A GIFT OF HEART

INSPIRING TRUE STORIES ABOUT HEART DOCTORS, PATIENTS AND SURGERIES

LINGARAJ NATH

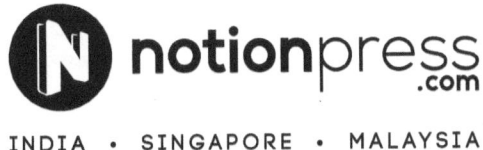

INDIA • SINGAPORE • MALAYSIA

Notion Press

No.8, 3rd Cross Street
CIT Colony, Mylapore
Chennai, Tamil Nadu – 600004

First Published by Notion Press 2021
Copyright © Lingaraj Nath 2021
All Rights Reserved.

ISBN 978-1-63669-688-1

This book has been published with all efforts taken to make the material error-free after the consent of the author. However, the author and the publisher do not assume and hereby disclaim any liability to any party for any loss, damage, or disruption caused by errors or omissions, whether such errors or omissions result from negligence, accident, or any other cause.

While every effort has been made to avoid any mistake or omission, this publication is being sold on the condition and understanding that neither the author nor the publishers or printers would be liable in any manner to any person by reason of any mistake or omission in this publication or for any action taken or omitted to be taken or advice rendered or accepted on the basis of this work. For any defect in printing or binding the publishers will be liable only to replace the defective copy by another copy of this work then available.

Dedication

To

My wife Archeeta

And

My children Navya and Nihira

CONTENTS

Foreword	7
1. Bajrangi's Tale	11
2. A Gift from the Heart	19
3. Turn the Clock Back	95
4. Angels of the Heart	181
Acknowledgment	249
Notes	251

FOREWORD

Every conversation starts from the heart. To have a conversation about heart is a unique situation!

For centuries, the heart was considered traditionally as a repository of "the soul". It was, therefore, considered a no-go zone for surgeons. Many even believed it as unethical to challenge any flaw in the heart as it was what "the Creator and almighty" himself wanted; be it a baby with congenital malformation of the heart or a young man suddenly succumbing to a heart attack. The flaws were in us to bear and accept.

Sometime in the second decade of twentieth century, the status quo on heart disease and treatment started to shift. A few brave-hearted doctors started going against the flow and toiling hard to give healing touch to babies and adults suffering from heart problems. They were no ordinary men or women.

Many of these heart-healers were stubborn eccentrics, many others geniuses with dexterous fingers, some were megalomaniacs, and a few were egocentric to the level of having a generational feud. However, each one of them had "one common goal"; to achieve success in an unexplored field and give life to people till now considered as "hopeless cases". Going through their life stories is not only a tale of thrilling medical history but is also a journey cutting across personal weakness or racial prejudices and achieving miracles in the face of adversity.

As I stand and watch inside the operation theater of the cardiac surgery wing, my fellow surgeon is busy in cutting and stitching the parts of a heart to insert an artificial valve in place of a defunct natural one. An open-heart surgery is in progress. When I look further into the chest the heaving and beating great organ is lying motionless, supported by a modern heart-lung machine while the surgeon and his team are repairing the problem.

To my surprise, there is no tension or wrinkled foreheads in anybody's face; even the chief surgeon gets time to remember and plan about the upcoming birthday of his first OT assistant. The procedure goes on in a fairly comfortable and routine manner and is later completed with a success. Today a typical heart surgery can be expected to have a success rate comparable to any other surgeries of the human body.

This success and predictability in complex cardiac surgery were achieved by the generations of cardiac surgeons who would not be afraid to come to the operation theater knowing the death rate was as high as 60-70%. These fearless doctors built brick by brick often spending an entire lifetime to create the modern-day edifice of heart surgery.

Today, when I talk to many patients who have had a valve replaced, a bypass surgery done or a pacemaker implanted, it is always a wonder to me. It reminds me about the trials and tribulations the first surgeons faced and the massive risk of almost certain death the early patients subjected themselves to while undergoing surgeries. What I could not tell these lucky patients probably finds a place in the following pages. The unique stories of creation of each of the procedures are very recent; most cardiac innovations are less than five decades old.

Is the person heart-dead or brain-dead …is a curiously strange question to ask. Everybody knows a person is dead when the heart stops. How does it matter which one stops first, the heart or the brain? The semantics would look ridiculous had it not been the entire medicolegal authenticity of heart transplant and many other organ transplants being critically dependent on them. The pioneers just dared to "switch hearts" in a daring surgery without any legislation to back them. With that, history was made and soon the legislations to define brain-death were ushered in. Laws and social norms have often juggled to go along medical innovations coming at breathtaking speed.

Today heart disease is the "no. 1 killer" in any society. Every third person is going to have cardiac ailment in his lifetime and every fourth person will be a victim and succumb due to heart problem. I am often asked if heart disease will ever be defeated. Nobody has the answer to the question yet. If the energy, perseverance and success against adversity of early pioneers of heart doctors are taken as the yardstick, there is definitely hope for humanity.

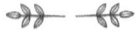

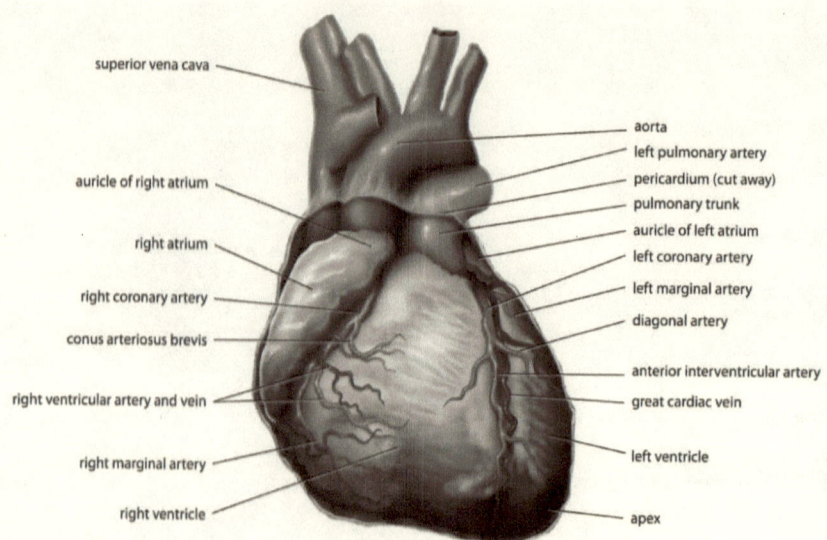

The Heart

CHAPTER 1

BAJRANGI'S TALE

*"Hold fast to dreams, For if dreams die
Life is a broken-winged bird, That cannot fly."*

— **Langston Hughes**

*"Hope
Smiles from the threshold of the year to come,
Whispering 'it will be happier'..."*

— **Alfred Lord Tennyson**

Within the deep jungles and hilly terrains of Odisha's backward areas, Bolangir is a small mofussil town. The city, if it can be called so, has no reason to exist except for the basic utilitarian purpose of supply of a few essentials which the nearby tribals and villagers cannot produce for themselves. The difficult landscape leaves people with very few opportunities other than basic subsistence-level agriculture. The only job-creating unit, a highly secretive ordnance factory, is present a few miles away from the city producing ammunition for the Indian army; probably established as a strategic reason of inaccessibility.

I reached Bolangir that morning after a hectic twelve-hour overnight train journey passing through one of the most beautiful landscapes and crossing a state border. The purpose of my journey was to attend a medical camp. A voluntary organization, who takes care of patients with heart disorders, had organized the medical program after three months of proper planning and tiresome effort coordinating with our hospital. They had chosen Bolangir as the venue as this place had no cardiologists or cardiac surgery facilities anywhere within or nearby.

After reaching the railway station, I was welcomed by Durgaprasad, one of the organizers. Durgaprasad took me to a nearby guesthouse for refreshment and later accompanied me to the camp venue.

As soon as we reached the camp, I met with an unexpected scene. I was expecting just a handful of patients, but the place was overflowing with crowds spilling out of the clinic! Some patients, with their relatives, were even sitting on the roads waiting for their turn. I couldn't understand why they had kept so many patients in the camp as each patient with a cardiac problem needs to be observed in detail as a new workup.

I looked at Durgaprasad and asked, being sarcastic. "There is a whole village here for medical check-up." He flashed a big smile at me and said, "Sir, our their team had made announcements on bullock carts all around the nearby villages for the last fifteen days about the upcoming camp. It is so nice and successful."

In fact, Durgaprasad was expecting to be congratulated for his effort. I had no answer to this logic. Anyway, I started my checkup and observed the patients minutely.

While some hours into the work, suddenly I heard a commotion outside my clinic room. The buzz was so much I couldn't control myself, and I immediately called the attendant to ask what the issue was.

"One minute. Give space please." The attendant and health camp assistant's voice were tense and face dark with worry as they pushed people away from the entrance to create a path. Soon the attendant came into my chamber with in a small baby accompanied by its parents. The baby was only eighteen days old! As small and fragile as a baby can be, the child was also extremely underweight.

I immediately got up to have a careful look. I could barely see the small frame of his body visible under the clothes. His eyes looked staring and his skin pale blue. For a moment I did not know what to do. In the large multispecialty hospital where I work, such sick patients never come to the Outpatient Department. They are immediately wheeled to intensive care from the Emergency Department with oxygen support. The nearest hospital being 400 km away, I had no option but to examine the child.

The heavy suffered breathing and heaving chest of the child was very significant the moment I lifted his clothes. With each breath, all the chest muscles of the child were trying frantically to take in whatever oxygen it could from the room air. There was a clear sign that he had a cardiac problem from birth.

To be confirmed of my diagnosis, "I immediately took him for an echocardiogram in a makeshift ultrasound machine". In the grainy pictures of the old out-of-age machine, I could decipher a problem. The aortic valve, which separates the lower pumping chamber from the great vessel aorta supplying blood to the body, looked very thick and over-bright, reflecting ultrasonic waves back to the transducer and was visible on the screen. The aortic valve leaflets of the baby's heart had fused to each other in thick fibrous strands, letting them barely move. It was a diagnosis of congenital stenosis of the aortic valve.

When I took hemodynamic measurements, they were even worse. The amount of blood allowed to pass from the left ventricle to the aorta through the aortic valve was "barely a fraction" of what is needed to sustain life. The problem had probably started while the baby was in utero. To be precise, it was a congenital deformity of the heart. Hence, the difficult part of counseling and explaining the problem to the parents began right at that very moment. I took them to my chamber, and then I explained to them about the problem as much as I could with the help of a diagram. I also let them know one terrible truth. This variety of congenital problems of the heart is described in medical books as "critical aortic stenosis" and is one of the most unforgiving conditions affecting babies. The lower chamber of the heart, which pumps blood through the malfunctioning aortic valve to the body, had dilated and was already contracting up to a third less than what it should in a normal baby. If the obstructed valve is not released within thirty days of delivery, the heart will go into irreversible failure. After the damage to the left ventricle at the end of thirty days, no treatment will ever be able to correct the problem leading to "an endless spiral to death."

As I grimly went through the records, I observed that the baby had already passed "eighteen days" of the tight timeline. In a modern hospital, these babies are taken for surgery right at birth. In fact, some cardiac centers with excellent neonatal heart-care team go a step forward to operate the baby while still in the mother's womb. By a specialized ultrasound test called fetal echocardiogram, such a condition is diagnosed before birth.

Once diagnosed, with the mother under general anesthesia, a needle and catheter are passed through the uterus of the mother and then onto the fetal heart. The main focus of this in-utero-intervention is to operate the stenotic aortic valve. This is basically conducted with the help of a balloon catheter before there is any negative effect on the growth of the left ventricle. A left ventricle with more adequate size and function may be present at birth if there is a chance of restoration of the normal blood flow.

I glanced at the baby's parents and saw their eyes filled with hope. "I explained to them the need for a balloon aortic valve surgery as soon as possible which could be done only in a big city like Bangalore or Delhi". They looked at me and asked a few more questions which I answered. I sent them off after explaining again. But I already believed in my mind that the baby would be dead soon as it happens to thousands of babies with heart defects born each year in India's hinterland.

Since then, five years had passed. I had, in the meantime, changed my job and was working in a different city in another larger referral hospital. One day while I was sitting in my OPD, a child walked into my room with his parents. He was wearing a colorful ethnic dress of the western Odisha people. Before I could ask anything, the father brought out the crumpled old prescription from his file. It was my handwritten diagnosis and advice for the same child back from the health camp! I could barely believe it and went on rubbing my eyes in disbelief.

"What is your name?" I asked the child.

"Bajrangi," he said, almost in a whisper.

Most Indian babies are named after a certain period after birth, as the parents think it inauspicious to name babies before or immediately at birth probably knowing the slim chance of survival to adulthood in most poor communities. The parents had named Bajrangi after the great Indian God Hanuman, who is known to have extraordinary powers and achieved many miracles in the mythology of Ramayana. The family elders possibly hoped that some of the miracles would be rubbed off on him too!

Bajrangi's father told me the entire story. After I left, the family had a discussion. They arranged money by selling family ornaments and mortgaging land for arranging the airfare and reached Bengaluru's Narayana Hrudayalaya Hospital. There, Bajrangi was admitted and underwent balloon valvoplasty surgery on an urgent basis as there was hardly any time to spare. In the Cath Lab, the doctors passed a tiny 4-mm balloon through Bajrangi's groin artery up to the heart. Once positioned across the valve, the balloon was inflated with guided pressure to crack open the fused valve leaflets to let the blood flow out of Bajrangi's heart into the aorta and general circulation. After the operation was over, his color and growth came back to normal. Six months after successful surgery and discharge Bajrangi was given his name in a small ritual ceremony at home.

Now, after five years, he looked absolutely normal with chubby cheeks and a shy smile on his face. As I looked at Bajrangi in wonder, he came forward to clasp me in a hug. Probably his parents had told him many stories about me. More than that I liked to believe he felt that intuitively in himself.

After they left, I couldn't stop thinking about Bajrangi. **In this universe, even without our knowing, lives are often connected by coincidences and miracles.** What if I had not gone to that remote place that day or was delayed by a month? And what if Bajrangi's father had missed that "bullock cart announcement" about the cardiac camp being conducted by the voluntary group? Without a chance diagnosis and advice from me and the leap of faith taken by the parents rushing for surgery by marshaling all their resources, Bajrangi would not have made it beyond a few months of painful existence and suffering. I also could not help being amazed by the wondrous miracles of medical science which has given life to such near-impossible cases. If all goes well, Bajrangi would live a normal lifespan with a good education and everything.

However, this was not always like this. Happy endings were unlikely with most kids with similar problems. In the long history of medical science spanning a few millennia, heart surgery remained as one of the last riddles to be solved.

The first artificial valve was implanted only about sixty years back. Most of the other developments in cardiac surgery and medicine have happened only over the last century. In a matter of a few decades, the treatment has changed which did not happen in five thousand years. Most of these developments have been through a series of miracles and chance happenings, but always anchored by the firm conviction and hard work of the pioneers. Bajrangi is the "poster-boy" of the success of heart surgery and this process of evolution.

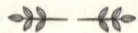

CHAPTER 2

A GIFT FROM THE HEART

"You give but little when you give of your possessions. It is when you give of yourself that you truly give."

– Kahlil Gibran

"The meaning of life is to find your gift. The purpose of life is to give it away."

– Pablo Picasso

Living On Borrowed Time

Cape Town, South Africa, during December is a wonderful destination for all travel-lovers. The holiday spirit is in full swing at this time of the year. Being located in the southern hemisphere, December is "the sunniest month" of the year. Cape Town also is famous for having longer days, glorious sunshine and divine natural beauty to attract tourists from all across the world. Other famous things about Cape Town are long and beautiful, serene beaches, which are frequented by locals and foreigners alike during these times. If one goes a little further within the inlands, the beautiful and unique "table mountain" is visible, standing majestically in the backdrop of the greens.

On this particular fateful day of December, however, it was gloomy and dull. The eventful day unfolded not on the beaches or mountains but in the dull gray university hospital building of Groote Schuur Hospital of Cape Town. It was always in the cardiac ward of the clinical wing where the "most serious" of heart ailment patients were admitted for treatment. Lying on one of the beds was a fifty-four-year frail man, staring impassively out of the windows. His name was Mr. Louis Washkansky. A forlorn aura hung around him.

Louis Washkansky has been helplessly bedridden for his "heart trouble" for a very long time. This Cape Town resident, Lithuanian-Jewish migrant's eyes vividly reflected his despondency and hopelessness. Prolonged illness and repeated hospitalization had sapped his energy away. On top of this, recently his investigation reports had been handed over to his doctors. He was told by the doctors of Groote Schuur Hospital that "he would certainly not survive to see the next winter, if not earlier".

At that time, it was December 2 in the year 1967 in South Africa. Racial segregation against blacks was ongoing and so was the resistance to apartheid. In the very same year in March, the African National

Congress and the Zimbabwe African People's Union formed an alliance for armed struggle against South Africa and Rhodesia. South Africa had been banned from various sports organizations like the Commonwealth Games and Tokyo Olympics by the international communities. Overall, the racial tension and subsequent economic issues made South Africa remain in not one of the best of its times. But all this mattered little at the moment to Washkansky who was fighting the monster of illness since the last few mundane years.

Louis Washkansky was born in the year 1914 in Kovno (today Kaunas), Lithuania. When he was nine years of age, his mother took him and his three siblings to Cape Town. There they were united with their father. He had come earlier so that they could have the means to survive happily and have a new home. A few years after completing his school studies, Washkansky joined the army for serving the country. Washkansky was indulged in active service during World War II in the East and North Africa and Italy. He also was an avid sportsman. He took part in football, swimming, and weightlifting. After the war came to an end, Washkansky returned to Cape Town and opened his own grocery. He married Anne Sklar, who was also a child immigrant in South Africa hailing from Lithuania. He had a lovely normal life, but "capricious destiny wanted differently".

Soon afterward, Washkansky's health declined substantially. He was diabetic and soon developed an incurable heart disease. He majorly suffered from three consecutive heart attacks. The last of these heart attacks was severe and led to congestive heart failure and cardiomyopathy. This is a condition of the heart when the capacity of the heart to pump blood becomes severely impaired.

A normal human heart has a "conical screwing motion" by which the blood is effectively pushed from apex to the base and finally to the aorta to be circulated in the body smoothly. But in patients with cardiomyopathy and heart failure, the heart becomes dilated excessively. It looks like a spherical balloon filled with excess fluid that keeps quivering aimlessly.

And the pumping is ineffective resulting in most of the blood to remain within the heart itself. Because of reduced blood supply, the vital organs like the brain, the kidneys, and the liver start to malfunction. Washkansky would often feel dizzy and fatigued. A very short walk to the toilet would make him struggle to "gasp" for breath. His legs and abdomen would swell up and his face would become pale and dry, giving an ashen look. When he was observed at Groote Schuur Hospital, his heart was seen to pump only one-third of the required blood. Washkansky had become invalid and unable to do any meaningful work.

In April 1966, Washkansky visited Groote Schuur Hospital. Doctors first performed several laboratory tests and an in-depth examination of Washkansky's condition and came to the conclusion that his situation was indeed serious. Due to the persistently failing heart, Washkansky was referred to Mervyn Gotsman, a cardiologist at the Cardiac Clinic in Groote Schuur Hospital, in the year 1967 in January. Washkansky underwent a critical cardiac catheterization and the observations confirmed severe heart failure. He was subsequently discharged after prolonged treatment.

Unfortunately, this was not the end of the agony. Washkansky had to be re-admitted in Groote Schuur on September 14, 1967, which was also the much-awaited Jewish New Year. He had gone down further clinically by the time. Once he became unconscious, which was found to be a diabetes coma. Most other times he was swollen with fluid accumulating inside his body and was in considerable pain. His wife Ann was always beside him and went to every extent to take care of him properly.

Washkansky knew he had only a small glint of hope left for him. Life was ebbing away, and he could do nothing other than praying to the Almighty. He was expecting with all his power that his doctor would bring some good news for him soon. On one fine day, which would become a landmark in his life, he was sent to meet the cardiac surgeon of Groote Schuur Hospital Dr. Christiaan Barnard.

***

Dr. Christiaan Barnard was a capable cardiothoracic surgeon from Cape Town Hospital and Heart Center. This tall and handsome white man's aura and confident manner created a great impression on Washkansky on the very first visit. The affable surgeon was Chief of experimental surgery as well as Associate Professor at Cape Town University. He was passionate about new heart surgery techniques. He had been working in the field of experimental as well as clinical heart surgery in South Africa for the last few years. After completing his medical training Barnard had gone to the United States to work at the University of Minnesota, Minneapolis. The cardiac department at Minneapolis was led by the pioneering heart surgeon Dr. Walton Lillehei. After returning from the USA, Barnard focused on developing the cardiac center of Groote Schuur Hospital. Though he had developed a good practice and had become a competent surgeon, he was not very well known outside his circle of hospital and community. But things would change soon. Christiaan Barnard would soon be described by people as "charismatic, youthful, compassionate, humanistic, and an energetic team leader".

Barnard was not the kind of person who would take a 'no' for an answer even when facing an adversary like destiny. Like a true surgeon, he always believed that anything wrong in the human body can be corrected by "gifted" surgical procedures. It is only that we have not achieved them yet. We still could muster the courage to try a bit more. This ever-smiling and affable surgeon had the habit of taking the most difficult clinical challenges and search for some solution.

One such challenge was for the heart patients like Washkansky, the clinical stage which was then called irreversible or end-stage heart failure. This actually meant that the patient's heart due to various causes like diabetes, high blood pressure, excessive alcohol consumption or infection would fail to maintain proper circulation and would not be able to work as an expert pump, which is the primary function of the heart as an organ. In Washkansky's case, it was the diabetes and smoking which probably did him in. Since there was no specific treatment or surgery for this, these patients would be prescribed a few medicines and would be asked to take bed-rest for most periods of life. These poor souls would remain mostly bedridden at home or end up spending months in the hospital every now and then. This would be the prolonged painful journey of these patients' lives, till the time the heart would give up. Doctors could do very little to change the course of illness, no matter what they tried. Many of these patients would develop psychological issues like depression, loneliness, or anxiety. Many even chose the path of suicide knowing the inevitable fate awaiting them at the other end of this dark tunnel of life, in which they were helplessly imprisoned.

Going against the prevalent mainstream scientific thought, Christiaan Barnard believed that there is indeed a treatment for such patients. Since the chambers of the heart had dilated severely and irreversibly, he guessed a practical solution would be to replace the existing heart with a new "donor-heart". His stint in the USA where already a lot of research was going on in this field convinced him of that. **It was just an arrangement of destiny that Washkansky suffering from a similar ailment would land in Christiaan Barnard's clinic.**

When Barnard started taking interest in developing a newer surgical technique, cardiac surgery was taking "baby steps from the centuries of slumber". A renowned British surgeon, Stephen Paget, made a statement in his textbook on "Surgery of the Chest" earlier in the year 1896. "Surgery of the heart has probably reached the limit set by nature to all surgery; no new method and no new discovery can overcome the natural difficulties that attend a wound of the heart." In the same year, however, a stab wound of the heart was successfully repaired by Ludwig Rehn of Frankfurt. Hence, the era of cardiac surgery had begun.

Cardiac surgery lagged behind other surgeries because of the sheer risk and complexity involved in tackling an organ through scalpels and sutures; that too an organ which was in motion in perpetuity throwing out more than three hundred liters of blood every hour.

It was during World War II when with the earlier advent of penicillin and better sterilization, cardiac surgery truly started to grow. The performance of extracardiac procedures began with the ligation of a persistent patent ductus arteriosus by Robert E. Gross in 1938. During the 1940s came Clarence Crafoord's repair of aortic coarctation, a procedure by which the narrowing of the aorta, which is the major artery of the heart, was corrected. The Blalock-Taussig procedure done at Johns Hopkins Hospital became useful for relieving the effects of hypoxia and polycythemia in the cyanotic congenital condition called tetralogy of Fallot. In England, Russell C. Brock relieved pulmonic stenosis in three patients who had tetralogy of Fallot, reducing the right-to-left intracardiac shunting.

But unlike the heart diseases mentioned previously, no such hope had been given out to patients like Washkansky suffering from a heart condition known as cardiomyopathy with severe ventricular dysfunction. During the 1960s, the global thought of the treatment of an irreversibly damaged heart, for various reasons like ischemic or congenital cardiomyopathy, was to take medicines and to be bedridden to avoid exertion. They were like basket cases hoping to survive for a few months or years in a nonfunctional state.

On the day Barnard had the fateful encounter with Washkansky, he elaborately explained the possibility of a transplant to him. Barnard explained to Washkansky that "his heart was not pumping enough for its long-term survival". He also told him that all other treatment approaches for him had been exhausted, and the only option left for Washkansky was a transplant. **To put it simply, Washkansky was to receive a heart from another person in place of his malfunctioning heart.** Washkansky and his wife Ann were just too struck with astonishment to give any reply in return. Their simple brains could not understand such complicated details. Barnard also explained to them that this operation had not yet been performed "anywhere in the world". He concluded by requesting permission to proceed from both of them on behalf of his surgical team and Groote Schuur Hospital.

Barnard had told them the whole truth. In 1967, a heart transplant was indeed new and was the most innovative experimental surgery. If successful, the operation would create "the world's first" and most glorious turn in the history of medical science. Not only would the operation save Washkansky's life, but it would also give hope and courage to many other heart patients and cardiac surgeons all over the world to offer the operation to their patients, for whom the alternative is certain death within days or months.

But heart transplant in the 1960s was a daunting task. Many surgeons had contemplated the procedure, but nobody had dared to proceed with the surgery. Compared to the recent available medical facilities and technologies, operative standards at that time were very primitive. The first obstacle to this was, of course, getting a donor. To be a donor, a person must be declared clinically brain-dead but must be having a well-functioning heart at the same time. This was a rare occurrence. The legal aspects of declaring a patient brain-dead when the heart would still be pumping were not yet initiated. Like in many aspects of research and scientific discovery concerning social norms, the relevant laws would be framed afterward.

A scientific panel committee at Harvard Medical School published a pivotal 1968 report to define irreversible coma. "The Harvard criteria" eventually and gradually gained consensus toward what is in recent times called brain-death. In the wake of the 1976 Karen Ann Quinlan case, state legislatures in the United States moved to accept brain-death as an acceptable indication of death. All this happened in later years. But in Washkansky's case, taking the heart of a patient for the purpose of a transplant was a gray-zoned idea fraught with medicolegal uncertainty.

Also, there was the issue of getting a person to agree to undergo such a complex surgery that was never attempted before. "To completely remove his own heart and put in its place a donor heart was an unthinkable idea". This had to be done while maintaining the blood circulation in the body by a heart-lung perfusion bypass machine, within a very short time.

Third and the most difficult part of the course was that no doctor in the world at that time knew how the donated heart would behave in the new body, and if the receiving body would accept or reject the precious graft.

Washkansky, however, quickly agreed to the possibility. He was by now already a hopeless man who would even clutch to a floating straw as a chance. As Barnard would himself describe afterwards "He was like a man chased by lions facing a river swamped with crocodiles. He would jump into the river hoping that somehow he could swim across without being savored by the crocodiles." Ann, his wife, told to an interviewer how Washkansky became very positive and excited while describing the possibility with their family members.

After Washkansky and his family gave their consent, Barnard told his hospital team to look for a suitable donor for the heart transplant. He also started to prepare himself and his team for this important procedure. Already Barnard had an experimental lab where animal experiments on transplant in canine models were being practiced. All the physiological findings and follow-ups of animal surgeries were meticulously recorded. Besides what he needed was an excellent and trusted team of associate surgeons. He knew that his team must have experienced anesthetists, pathologists, and immunologists besides a good group of technicians and nurses. Barnard discussed the issue with his team including his younger brother Maurius Barnard, who was also a cardiac surgeon at Groote Schuur Hospital. Barnard was confident that they had a good chance of success. However, at that moment the main problem for him was getting a suitable donor for Washkansky.

An opportunity finally came for Washkansky in November 1967. A young black man had met with a catastrophic road accident. He had badly injured his brain due to a serious head injury. When he was admitted to Groote Schuur Hospital, no signs of neurological activity were found. His family was approached for heart donation after neurosurgeons declared his case as "non-salvageable". However, the electrocardiogram taken after the accident showed significant ischemic changes in the young man. It meant that his heart might have possibly been damaged due to a reduced oxygen supply. The transplant was hence canceled much to Washkansky's disappointment. He had been cleaned and shaved for the procedure. For him, it was a big letdown. He had no option but to wait and hope for better luck next time.

***

Miracle At Midnight

"A remarkable though tragic thing happened a few days later as if by providence." On Saturday, December 2, 1967, Denise Darvall, a beautiful girl aged twenty-five years, had gone to the main road in the observatory of Cape Town market for buying a cake along with her mother. While crossing the road, a standing truck blocked Denise and her mother's vision from upcoming traffic. A pick van was approaching them at high speed. The drunk driver skipped the traffic light and hit Denise and her mother who were in the middle of crossing the road.

In split second, both Denise and her mother were thrown across the road. Denise's mother died instantly on the spot. Denise sustained a skull fracture and severe head injuries after the car flung her across the road; her head hit the wheel cap of the car. She was immediately wheeled by paramedics to Groote Schuur Hospital. She required life support to remain alive and thus was essentially "brain-dead" by the time she made it to the hospital. At around 9 P.M. on the day of the accident, the resuscitation team had to stop every attempt to revive her.

Edward Darvall, Denise's father rushed to the hospital upon getting this dreadful news. He was absolutely shattered seeing his dead wife and critically ill daughter. The 66-year-old Edward was also given a sedative, and he waited while the doctors attempted to save his daughter.

Afterward, when Darvall regained proper consciousness, he wanted to know about the condition of his daughter. Two doctors, Coert Venter and Bertie Bosman, informed him that there was nothing further they could do for Denise. But Bosman also explained to him that there was a man in the hospital who they might be able to help and asked Edward if he would consider allowing them to "transplant Denise's heart".

It was a moment of deep tragedy for Edward Darvall. He excused himself from the doctors to have some alone time. The doctors also told him he may take whatever time he required and wanted him to decide freely as they did not want him to feel forced. But surprisingly, Edward came out in only four minutes to meet them. He had composed himself and made up his mind. He had taken the decision to give permission for the donation of Denise's heart.

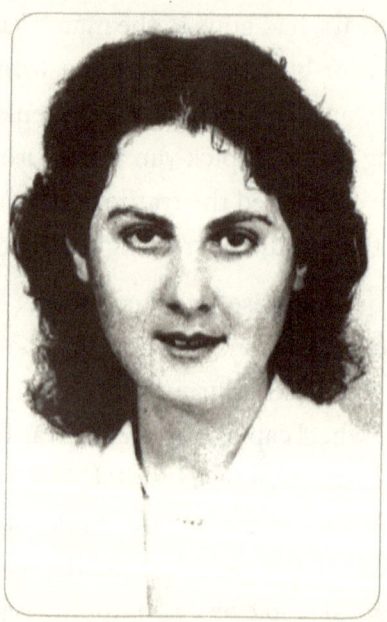

FIG: Denise Darvall. She was "the donor" in the world's first successful human heart transplant, performed at Groote Schuur Hospital, South Africa, by a team of surgeons led by Christiaan Barnard.

It was magnificently generous of Denise's father to give consent for the surgery. Back in 1967, hardly any awareness about organ transplants was there among the public. To give up his loving daughter's heart before burial would have meant a lot to Edward. He later told that his daughter was carrying a birthday cake for him, there was a heart design on it where it was written *"Daddy we love you"*. Also, Denise had received her first salary recently and bought gifts for her family members. Since she was so giving always, Edward said, "It was only fitting that her heart would be donated to save someone's life." Often it happens that one person's tragedy is another one's hope. **This magnificent gesture of Mr. Edward staged the set for Washkansky's surgery, an event which will be written forever in golden letters in medical history.**

It was late in the night when Barnard's phone rang in his house. It had been frustrating for Mr. Barnard to have been waiting for so long for a suitable donor for Washkansky's transplant. He was informed that a donor-heart has become available. Barnard immediately asked the nurse to alert his team, consisting of approximately thirty people and himself, to arrange for the operation.

***

The operation began at the stroke of midnight and continued till morning. The nurses had prepared two operating tables in the adjoining rooms. One for Mr. Washkansky, the recipient, and one for Miss Denise, whose heart would be donated. At that time, there was no clear legislation of declaring a patient dead in South Africa. The law simply stated that "a patient was considered dead when he or she was declared dead by two physicians". There was no mention of brain-death or stoppage of heart as criteria for declaring a patient as dead. Therefore, it was Barnard who concluded that he could simply use the term brain-death as a criterion for properly declaring a patient's death. Barnard also invited a local medical examiner to be present during the surgery as a precaution. The examiner would be a witness and concur to the fact that Denise had indeed been declared dead when the transplant surgery of the donor-heart would take place. As a precaution, however, to avoid any possible medicolegal complications, he, later on, decided he would wait for the heart to stop beating before he removed it. He, therefore, disconnected the ventilator and waited until Washkansky's EKG showed no electrical activity at all. This took approximately six minutes.

After this, the surgeons began to operate on Denise. They split open her sternum to open up her chest. Her heart had stopped beating completely and was lying motionless. Without wasting much time, the surgical team connected her heart to a heart-lung machine. The perfusionist circulated cold oxygenated blood through her veins, with the aim of reducing the metabolism of the heart while it was waiting to be transplanted. The heart was then cooled to a low temperature instantly, which helped in protecting it from further ischemic injury during the time of the transplantation.

The donor-heart was excised cautiously in such a manner that the portion of atria and the four pulmonary veins draining into it would be left behind. In a similar manner afterward, Washkansky's heart too would be dissected so that his portions of the right and left atriums and veins will be left behind. This was intended to make the surgery less complicated and avoid causing four extra-venous anastomoses of the pulmonary veins. This surgery was earlier practiced in the animal lab on dogs by Barnard and his younger brother and fellow cardiac surgeon Maurius Barnard several times. This part of the surgery went smoothly. However, some "serious trouble" waited for the team in the other room, when the heart transplant was finally about to take place.

Barnard was busy in the meantime working on Washkansky's transplant procedure. He waited till the heart from Denise was successfully harvested. Then he cut open Washkansky's chest and did a delicate job of removing the diseased heart. It was very big and disfigured suffering from years of insults. When the heart was removed, it left a huge space inside Washkansky's chest. Looking at the cavernous space for a moment Barnard thought for a moment if the relatively small organ of Denise's heart would do the job. The importance of the event came upon him to the fullest extent. **Even though he had done hundreds of heart surgeries in his life, this was certainly unique.**

The donor-heart was quickly sewn in place without difficulty, after putting stitches to the posterior surface of the heart at the atrial chamber where the four pulmonary veins enter the heart. Thereafter, the two major outlet arteries, aorta and pulmonary artery, were stitched in to complete the transplant. The next step was the gradual warming of the heart to bring it to the normal temperature.

The very moment Barnard was done with the transplant procedure, he allowed the blood to perfuse through the new heart from the recipient's heart-lung machine. While doing this, he also raised the patient's body temperature to normal by continuously warming the blood as it passed through the heart-lung machine. The surgical team waited with bated breath for the heart to start beating. But the "newly transplanted" heart would not beat even after waiting for a few minutes, much to the dismay of everyone. Naturally, this increased Barnard's worries; he was thinking that the heart muscle had been damaged to a severe extent when he had to disconnect Denise's oxygen supply. He electrically defibrillated the heart with a 100-joule shock from the electric defibrillator. The team breathlessly watched when "Denise's heart started to beat slowly but surely inside Washkansky's chest". The electrocardiogram showing on the monitor began making beeping sounds on a regular pattern.

The problems were not over yet. The contractions of the new heart were very weak and could not take over the circulation properly. There was a problem somewhere. Barnard kept on double-checking each and every step for any mistakes, but there was none to be found.

Barnard tried twice to wean the patient from pump-oxygenator support, but the heart was not beating strongly enough to maintain adequate blood pressure. He had no other choice but to allow more time for the donor-heart to gain strength and continued to keep the patient alive on the heart-lung machine. After some time, they received some good results. The assistant informed Barnard that blood pressure was coming up. The perfusionist did another attempt at weaning from the heart-lung machine. This time, at the third attempt, he was successful. Pulse became steadier, saturation and other vitals remained intact. And finally, the moment came when Washkansky's new heart started to work independently without needing any support from the heart-lung machine.

Barnard felt a great relief on looking up at the monitor and Washkansky's face. He then looked around the room toward his team. That was a *eureka moment* for the whole team. At last, the moment arrived when the heart-lung machine could be switched off, and the chest was slowly closed. The operation had been successful with God's grace and the determination of the doctors. It had taken almost five hours to complete the whole procedure. It was 6:15 in the morning when the operation was over; the day was December 3, 1967. Barnard was now fully satisfied. He moved out of the room throwing the gloves into the waste bin and giving his assistants instructions to follow as he left the operation theater.

***

A Precious Gift

"Neither Dr. Barnard nor anybody else could ever dream of what would happen the next day". Barnard informed the superintendent of Groote Schuur Hospital, Dr. Jacobus Burger, about the surgery while exiting the hospital. From there, information was passed on to the local administrative unit of medical affairs at Cape Town. The news was found important enough to be passed on to the prime minister of South Africa. Within hours, the world got to know about the first heart transplant surgery—"the upcoming global sensation" just like the story of the first man stepping on the moon which would happen in the coming two years from that day. When in the afternoon Barnard returned to the hospital, the corridors were filled with journalists and television media people. The media took photographs of the whole team and interviewed them. **By the next morning, news of the first successful heart transplant in the world exploded into world news and television making gigantic headlines.** In today's scale, it would be termed as "going viral" or "to be the super trending news". Journalists and film crews kept flocking into Cape Town's Groote Schuur Hospital, in turn making Barnard and Washkansky the most famous household names.

The front page of *Cape Times*, the South African newspaper, captioned the news in bold as 'World's First Heart Transplant'. *Life Magazine* headlined the news with the caption 'A Gift of Heart' with a picture of a beaming Washkansky with two medical personnel on the front cover page. The sub-caption aptly read "A dying man lives with a dead girl's heart."

The reporting soon became as dramatic as the surgery itself. Initial reports widely hailed the operation as 'historic' and 'successful'. Unprecedented media attention for a medical undertaking was immensely attracted by the first heart transplant, ushering in a new era of postoperative press conferences, doctor and patient celebrities, and medical PR.

A news organization even ended up offering "one million dollars" to get a picture of the operation theater when Denise's heart was lowered into Washkansky. But they could not be obliged as there simply was no such picture taken. The reason was simple enough as Barnard had not thought of anything else other than achieving a successful result during the operation. He told afterward that he never expected it to become such an international phenomenon. Similarly, another newsgroup who hoped to pay and receive the famous gloves from the operating hands of Dr. Barnard was disappointed when they came to know he had discarded the gloves into the waste bin as this was his usual practice.

With this successful operation, the twentieth century found its most famous medical event. As reflected by one of the journalists, it had "everything a reporter could wish for." It was the most extraordinary technological feat involving the most iconic and precious human organ. **It became the ever-famous and intimate story of one young life lost allowing another to be saved.**

From his hospital ward, Washkansky's daily activities and emotions were reported in minute detail across the continents. Such trivial facts and tidbits of his life like "when he sat up, spoke, smiled, or even when he had a boiled egg for breakfast" were eagerly lapped up by the media. The public wanted to know everything about it, and Washkansky's life and daily living made front-page news almost every single day. Washkansky too was happy to oblige the media and the big politicians of the South African regime by allowing them to take his interview. The fame was not only of Washkansky's; his beloved wife and the donor's father were featured prominently in the media coverage as well. They were pictured together when Mrs. Washkansky was shedding tears of gratitude in front of Mr. Edward Darvall for agreeing to donate his precious daughter's heart, this precious 'gift of life'.

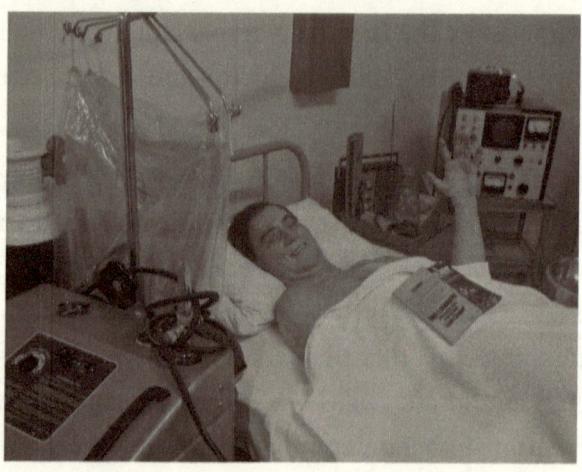

FIG: Louis Joshua Washkansky, a South African man who was the recipient of the "world's first human-to-human heart transplant".

Barnard, meanwhile, remained firmly in the limelight for a long time. He was only forty-five years of age at that time. But he handled the adulation and media pressure in a surprisingly calm and confident manner, like a complete professional. There would be a media briefing by Barnard about Washkansky's health and progress on a daily basis. This young and handsome doctor and his operation captured the public's imagination as no procedure had done before, and the personable Barnard within the blink of an eye became an international celebrity. Monarchs and Head of States honored him gratefully. According to French President Jacques Chirac, "Dr. Barnard will remain the symbol of audacious modern medicine, able to surpass accepted ideas to bring solutions to victims of suffering and illness." His photogenic and charismatic charm made him the perfect front-cover page, and he kept on appearing on magazine covers including the *Time* magazine as well. He met dignitaries and film stars, drawing crowds and photographers wherever he went. A private meeting with the Pope was arranged for him in Rome. He also made a highly published tour of the United States making an appearance on the CBS television show 'Face the Nation'. He had an audience with the President of the USA Mr. Lyndon B. Johnson. The media simply could not have enough of this "handsome and charismatic surgeon". They were completely mesmerized by his genius.

A few years later Barnard followed up his maiden heart transplant surgery with another feat. It happened by a chance discussion with a patient's relative. In 1973, Barnard performed a heart transplant in which the donor-heart failed to function satisfactorily. The patient died in the operating theater. When Barnard came out to break the sad news, he was asked "why he could not put the old heart back, as at least it had kept the patient alive". This struck Barnard as a distinct possibility. If the patient's own heart had been left in place, and the transplant was inserted as an auxiliary pump, failure of the donor-heart may not have caused the patient's demise.

To confirm the success of the proposal Barnard set up a research team to develop the surgical technique of "heterotopic heart transplantation" in the animal laboratory. The concept was for a second heart to be placed in the right chest and for the two hearts to function in parallel. Multiple techniques were tried in the lab and finally, a "piggy-back double-heart technique" was mastered after much experimentation. Soon Barnard proceeded with his novel heart transplant technique called heterotopic heart transplantation; the world's first such surgery whereby the original heart stays in-situ and a donor heart is put in another location most commonly in the right chest.

Forty-nine consecutive heterotopic heart transplants were performed in Cape Town between 1974 and 1983, the highest number of such cases anywhere in the world. Barnard came out with moderately good results for the cases; three of the first five patients, in fact, survived more than ten years. Afterward, with the introduction of the immunosuppressive therapies the incidence of sudden graft failure due to acute rejection decreased, thus eliminating one of the major advantages of heterotopic heart transplantation. Soon after heterotopic heart transplantation became less frequently used as a procedure compared to the routine orthotopic heart transplantation. The technique is still performed rarely at select transplantation centers, and indications include significant donor-recipient size mismatch or irreversible recipient pulmonary hypertension.

Medical historians were often unable to comprehend the reason for this outpouring of emotions, joy, and celebrations at the success of the first human-to-human heart transplant, also called orthotopic allograft. This was a thing discussed from the dinner table to the high society, analyzed by country heads to the medical fraternity. Everybody tried to discuss and express their feelings like it was in any way personally connected. **The amount of emotional outpouring the event created, crossing the national boundaries and racial divisions, was unique in the annals of medical history.**

After all these years, it can also be said that not even a single forward step in medical history can ever equal the heart transplant in kindling universal public interest to that extent. Within the blink of an eye, it became both a medical as well as media phenomenon; just as described by the *Daily Express* it was "the world's most talked-about operation." Likened to climbing Mount Everest or landing on the moon, this symbolic medical 'first' was straightaway incorporated into the chronicles of human achievement with much enthusiasm. Also, as the television was becoming available all around the world, the news was able to travel far and wide and was known to a greater number of people. People could see the live telecasts of events and people which even on black-and-white television screens had a far more emotional impact than reading in any newspaper. The "instant and cumulative effects" of media reports and imageries produced doctor and patient celebrities and made medical science exceptionally visible as a whole. Human history and its reporting had taken a brand-new turn.

One reason why Barnard made such an impact was that with this singular feat, he was able to break the mindset barrier of almost everyone around the world—an achievement, which can be considered as parallel like the "four-minute mile barrier" in athletics. Crossing the mile distance in under exactly four minutes was a dream that athletes had cherished for long. In this case, the runners had been chasing the goal diligently and seriously since the year 1886 at least, and that the challenge majorly involved Australia, Europe, and North America's most brilliant coaches and extremely talented athletes. All experts at that time had said that the human body physiologically lacked the capability of achieving the feat. It was too dangerous and unsafe to try.

For years athletes had been striving against the clock, but the elusive four minutes had always beaten them. Then also they never once gave up and their battle continued. To put it simply, it had become much of a "psychological barrier" than a physical one. Each and every time, the athletes would try their level best but would end up short of the target. Like an unconquerable mountain, the record stood untouched. Finally, Roger Banister, who on May 6, 1954, busted through the four-minute barrier with a time of three minutes, fifty-nine and four-tenths of a second. This changed a whole paradigm in the history of athletics bringing many more athletes across the elusive barrier. In the preparation for the run, Banister would, every day, think in his mind relentlessly of success to create a sense of certainty. He made it a daily routine in his practice and finally achieved the record in due time.

A similar thing was seen in the case of the heart transplant surgery. For years, surgeons and scientists all over the world had been dreaming of achieving the feat. But it was Barnard who finally, in that midnight feat of December 1967, made it an unexpected reality. After that, the path looked so much simpler. Surgeons since then acquired the confidence of experimenting with the most difficult and impossible surgeries. What followed was a brave new world of heart surgery open to any kind of experimentations breaking taboos and socio-religious barriers. All this was started by the diligent, hardworking, and valorous Dr. Christiaan Barnard, a remarkable surgeon with an even more arduous journey if looked from his humble origin to the "pinnacle of success".

***

Christiaan Barnard was born on November 8, 1922 in Beaufort West, a small country town in the Cape Province. Situated in the Great Karoo and approximately 300 miles away from Cape Town, the area around Beaufort can be mainly characterized as an arid region of scrub grassland where the major activity is sheep farming.

His father, Adam Barnard, was working at the Church. His earnings from the service rendered as pastor to mixed-race people were average, but he was an honest and hardworking person who managed to send all his children to college. According to him, "education was the most important part of life". In the year 1940, Barnard achieved his matriculation certificate from the Beaufort West High School. Then he decided to study medicine and got admitted to the University of Cape

Town Medical School. Here he successfully obtained his MB ChB in the year 1945.

It was his mother, Dr. Barnard often said, who instilled in him and his brothers the belief that they could do anything they set their minds to, and to top it all they could do it well. Young Christiaan successfully ran a record mile on his bare and scorched feet. He made his family proud by winning the school tennis championship though having a borrowed racquet and some mere cardboard covering the pitiful holes in his sneakers. He studied all alone under the rural firelight and then also was at the top of his class.

Barnard after finishing his basic medical course did his internship and residency at the Groote Schuur Hospital itself, after which he worked as a general practitioner in Ceres, a rural town within the Cape Province. In 1951, he decided to return to Cape Town. He worked at the City Hospital in the post of a Senior Resident Medical Officer, and in the Department of Medicine at the Groote Schuur Hospital mainly as a registrar where he did some research work on tubercular meningitis.

Barnard, along with the medical practice, also involved his evenings and night in the research work and animal experiments. By that time, he was married and also became a proud father. There were several difficulties that he had to face while running his household as well as his job with the research work. But Barnard would never stop his research work.

Initially, Barnard performed experiments on dogs while investigating intestinal atresia, a birth defect that allows life-threatening gaps to develop in the intestines. Many surgeons had tried to treat this condition, but no satisfactory method or result was found. He followed a medical hunch that this was caused by inadequate blood flow to the fetus. After nine months of hard work, he even was able to develop a cure for the condition mainly by removing that particular piece of the intestine with inadequate blood supply. To put it simply, the previous surgeons made a mistake of attempting to reconnect ends of the intestine; but this was not a good idea as these also had inadequate blood supply. To be successful, it was typically necessary to remove a longer length of the diseased intestine. This proved to be successful and in the later years got adopted by many other surgeons. Barnard got to publish and get noticed because of his extensive and elaborate research work. In 1953, he successfully completed his Master's degree, receiving a Master of Medicine from the University of Cape Town. In the same year, he also obtained a Doctorate in Medicine (M.D.) from the same university for a dissertation titled "The treatment of tuberculous meningitis."

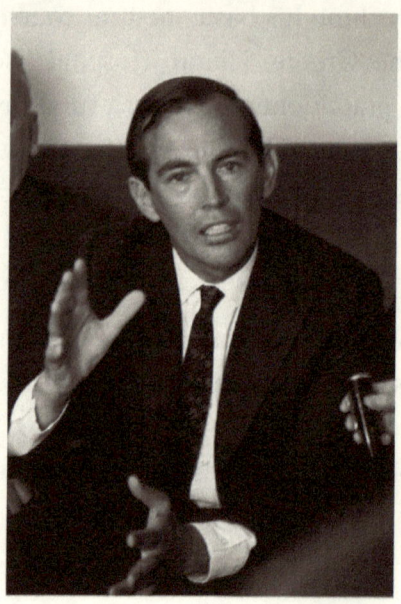

FIG: Christiaan Neethling Barnard, the South African cardiac surgeon who performed the world's first human-to-human heart transplant operation on December 3, 1967.

In 1955 he got an opportunity to go to Minneapolis, USA to study general surgery through a scholarship with Dr. Owen H. Wangensteen at the University of Minnesota. Barnard was overwhelmed to join there. But he was facing serious problems as the scholarship could barely cover his necessities. In his first few weeks there, he became so short of funds that—as he mentioned in an interview once—"he had to mow lawns, wash cars, and do many other such odd jobs to obtain his meal money".

Dr. Wangensteen assigned Barnard to work on gastrointestinal surgery cases. But the Almighty had different plans for the young Barnard. Whenever Barnard needed a break from this work, he frequently wandered across the hall to the nearby cafeteria. On one such day, he met Vince Gott who was the resident doctor with Dr. Walt Lillehei, the Chief Cardiac Surgeon of Minnesota University. Barnard and Gott developed good comradery through those meetings. Barnard accompanied Gott to attend cardiac surgery operations in his spare time. Dr. Lillehei was a pioneer and considered as the "Father of Open-Heart Surgery".

Lillehei's center at that time was one of the very few institutions of the world using a new technique of heart-lung machine for cardiac surgery. Gott used to assist Dr. Lillehei during his surgeries by reverse flow technique of running blood backward in the venous system. This was done mainly through the veins of the heart; as a result, Lillehei could simplistically and more easily perform an operation on the aortic valve. It was obvious that Barnard was deeply in love with cardiac surgery than gastrointestinal surgery. Then on a fateful day of March 1956, Barnard was asked by Gott to help him control the heart-lung machine for a certain operation. Shortly thereafter, Wangensteen agreed on letting Barnard switch to Lillehei's service. It was during this time that Barnard first became acquainted with the fellow surgeon Norman Shumway. This friendship was to have an ironic turn in the near future when Barnard would beat Shumway's team as well as another team from New York by a few days to be the first surgeon ever to do a successful human-to-human heart transplant.

Barnard bagged a degree in Master of Science in Surgery in the year 1958 for a thesis titled "The aortic valve – problems in the fabrication and testing of a prosthetic valve". That very same year he was also awarded a Ph.D. This was one of the most stimulating periods for Barnard as far as learning and research on novel cardiac surgery were concerned. He was happy to work under Cardiac Surgeon Lillehei and considered it the greatest learning of his career. Barnard described the two years he spent in the United States as "the most fascinating time in my life." Barnard worked hard in both the clinic as well as the research laboratory. Barnard was not the only one who praised Lillehei; the admiration was mutual. A few years later, particularly for Barnard's innovation, prodigious memory, courage, and seriousness as a scholar, Lillehei expressed his high regard for him. Lillehei noted that, although Barnard could be very charming, "He could provoke a rather intense dislike among some people—colleagues and staff—because he was always outspoken and often had unconventional ideas."

Lillehei offered Barnard a position in his team which was one of the most prestigious and respected cardiac teams in the world during those days. However, Barnard refused the offer at Minnesota. He wanted to come back to South Africa to provide service for his homeland. In 1958, he returned to South Africa from the United States.

As soon as Barnard returned to South Africa, he was appointed as the Head of the Department of Experimental Surgery at Groote Schuur Hospital, and he was also presented with a joint post at the University of Cape Town. He organized one of the first, and probably the best, open-heart surgery programs in Africa, working at both Groote Schuur and the nearby Red Cross Children's Hospital. Within a few years or so, this program acquired loads of success. It was recognized for its great progress in complex congenital heart surgery as well as for the continuous development of new techniques and technologies.

Barnard was a "thinker surgeon". Although not the most dexterous, he had excellent surgical judgment and the ability to obtain the results that he desired and aimed for. He was, however, prone to "outbursts of temper" when the procedure was not progressing smoothly according to his liking, and this trait antagonized several of his coworkers. But the team would still be together and functional primarily because at that time no group within the whole continent was doing anything more exciting than this. Cape Town's cardiac surgery program ranked high in the worldwide rankings. Several years earlier, before Barnard even performed the first heart transplant, he had already earned international recognition, particularly for achieving success in the repair of congenital anomalies.

In 1960, he was promoted to the post of full-time lecturer and Director of Surgical Research at the University of Cape Town. In the same year, he flew to Moscow to meet the great Russian surgeon Vladimir Demikhov. He was mainly known as "the foremost expert" in the field of organ transplants. It was during the Cold War Era and many of the medical achievements of Soviet doctors in those times were not well discussed within the western scientific community. Hence his research work was translated and appreciated much later by the scientists in the rest of Europe and America. Demikhov was an innovator in transplant surgery and was much ahead of many other European and American surgeons in the experimental surgery field. Barnard once said, "If there is a father of heart and lung transplantation then Demikhov certainly deserves this title."

In 1961, Barnard was appointed as the Head of the Division of Cardiothoracic Surgery at the teaching hospitals of the University of Cape Town. In the year 1962, within a very short span of time, he was able to rise to the position of Associate Professor in the Department of Surgery at the University of Cape Town. Barnard was then joined by Marius Barnard, his younger brother, who had also studied medicine. Together with Maurius as his capable assistant, Barnard developed a good team at the Department of Cardiac Surgery. After more than a thousand open-heart operations at GSH, Barnard's focus then shifted toward heart transplantation in the early 1960s.

***

I came to know about Neeraj's story in reverse: first about his present ill health and later about his life story. The first time I saw Neeraj, he was in ICU, unconscious and on ventilator support. Later I had a long chat with Neeraj one day while he was in the recovery ward of the cardiology wing in our hospital.

As a thirty-five-year-old handsome young man, he worked as a chartered financial analyst with five years of experience. He had a successful career working as a senior manager at a multinational business concern dealing with agricultural products. He was headquartered at Bhubaneswar; but as part of his job requirement, he had to travel from his posting place to various district-level zones on frequent intervals. He had married six months back. Then suddenly a couple of months back, he got a mail from New Zealand Immigration Office. It mentioned that his application for immigration to New Zealand had been approved. Overall, his life was on a roll.

Neeraj was elated about his long-cherished dream of relocating to New Zealand with his family. When Neeraj received the mail, he was at one of his outreaches works at the District Headquarter Kalahandi, a tribal interior place of Odisha. Neeraj wanted to finish his last-leg work and give notice to his employer farm when something "totally unexpected" happened to him.

Neeraj had traveled to a tribal interior place, situated within the faraway forest and hills 50 km from Kalahandi, on a field inspection work. Two days after returning, he came down with a bout of flu. He felt a vague body ache and had a runny nose for three days after which it subsided on its own. Neeraj had almost forgotten about it. But two weeks later while going on a morning walk, Neeraj felt unusually breathless, as if his legs were carrying extra weight. He stopped after a short distance and came back to his guest house.

The next morning, Neeraj noticed swelling around both his ankles. His abdomen felt bloated and he felt the flu had probably recurred. Since that was his last day at Kalahandi, Neeraj returned to Bhubaneswar with his driver where he planned to have a medical checkup after reaching home.

Neeraj's wife and parents received a call from an unknown number in the same evening; it was from the hospital. As the surprised family members rushed to the hospital, they found a seriously ill Neeraj on ventilator admitted in the ICU in the Cardiac Care Wing. The doctor on duty explained how "he was brought to emergency in a gasping condition, his mouth frothing with foamy secretion and severely low oxygen level". He was drowsy and incoherent due to the low level of oxygen his brain received. The doctors immediately intubated him and put on ventilator; further investigation and echocardiogram revealed he had developed severe heart failure. Both his cardiac chambers had swollen and enlarged massively. The pumping capacity of his heart was reduced to fifteen percent, the bare minimum to support life. The doctor asked the anxious relatives to meet me as I was the specialist in charge of treating Neeraj.

As the family met me at the consultation chamber, "anxiety was writ large on their faces". A healthy man on a business trip suddenly came down with a serious heart ailment; His family was eager to know how it happened. I told them it was cardiomyopathy, a condition affecting heart muscles. The damage can happen due to several causes such as viral infections, toxins, or metabolic factors. Many a time genetic factors may also be the culprit causing failing or poorly contractile heart. In Neeraj's case, given the history, it was possibly a case of "viral myocarditis"; a viral infection of the heart that started as innocuous flu symptoms a couple of weeks back when Neeraj was traveling to a distant forest area. Since he was put on ventilator with antibiotics and cardiac medications on the infusion pumps supporting his feeble heart, Neeraj's condition got stabilized and he showed signs of improving vitals. I told them that the current episode would improve; but the severe injury to cardiac muscles, which the viral-induced immune antibodies had caused, might be unfortunately irreversible in a significant percentage of cases. **It mostly depends on the amount of cardiac muscle cells destroyed by the immune attack converting them into worthless fibrous scar tissue.**

Since then, two and half months had passed already. I was attending a consultation session with Neeraj and his wife in my chamber. After the previous frantic presentation at emergency and later treatment in ICU he had been discharged one week later for a period of rest and medication.

Neeraj and his wife sat across my table, well dressed and elegant. From the looks of it, they might as well be mistaken for attending a routine consultation. However, both of them knew that something had irreversibly changed their life since the last episode when Neeraj was brought gasping and unconscious to the hospital emergency. The review of the echocardiogram had been done the previous day, and it showed his heart chambers grossly dilated and swollen with two major valves leaking blood backward with each cardiac contraction. Neeraj's heart was still as bad or probably worse than it was in the beginning. The medicines had drawn away extra fluid from his heart and circulatory system giving him physical relief. But the prognosis of his heart remained equally grim. Along with this, "his dream of emigration to New Zealand and starting a new life and career had also vanished". There was no way the immigration authorities would give Neeraj a medical fitness report. But these topics were never discussed. Neeraj's wife asked a few things about food and exercise, etc. when Neeraj brought up the topic himself.

"How about a heart transplant, doctor? I understand that this is a permanent damage to my heart muscles. What are the chances of success? And cost?" he asked.

A thing about the era of the Internet and Google Search is that doctors and patients have the same amount of knowledge to access about their disease. Only the perspective and approach differ from the point of view of a physician and a patient. Saying so, Neeraj lightened my burden with his research which he did while having his complete bed-rest for the last few months.

I agreed with his view that since twelve weeks had passed without any improvement of heart function, he was most likely to be in the category of irreversible cardiac failure also called "idiopathic dilated cardiomyopathy". On a medical management, the chance of long-term survival is grim, maybe less than a serious form of cancer in terms of five-year survival rate. I agreed that they may consult a transplant center for any further advice or listing to a transplant program. His wife, all this while, listened with silent attention; and I kept wondering what was going on in her mind. Neeraj left me thanking for all the care our team had given him. The very next day he flew to Hyderabad.

After four months, I met the transplant team cardiologist at Hyderabad at a conference. I asked him about Neeraj. As it turned out, Neeraj was evaluated by the team. He was found not yet at a stage where he would be offered a heart transplant as more severe symptomatic and eligible patients were on the queue. However, he would soon reach the stage given the poor function of his heart, the doctor agreed. Meanwhile, Neeraj was implanted with a pacemaker called ICD. This pacemaker can detect any electrical chaos and fibrillation inside the heart by an inbuilt computer algorithm analyzing the patient's heart rhythm and abort an episode of cardiac arrest. One of the ways how the poorly functioning hearts often end in sudden death. The pacemakers and other medications would work like a bridge till the time Neeraj became eligible for transplant and got a suitable donor.

***

Throughout the records of history and more so in medicine, the growth of human knowledge has been like "a series of strenuous stairs", each put up arduously by different persons. The stairs are connected by invisible threads. Scientists working at different times and space often would not know how all these will connect up. But it could well happen that over a period, one scientist from a particular country may use the path created by another. The end result at the summit is often a spectacular observation for the very last stage. The previous stages remain less visible though being equally valuable. Two such valuable scientific developments during the preceding period furthered the possibility of success in the heart transplant efforts of Dr. Barnard. One was the "cardiopulmonary bypass (CPB)" and the other was "hypothermia technique".

Cardiopulmonary bypass (CPB) is a basically technique in which a machine is temporarily made to take over the major function of the lungs and the heart during the surgery. This mainly helps in maintaining the oxygen content and the blood circulation of the patient's body. In fact, the CPB pump is itself often referred to as 'the pump' or a heart-lung machine. CPB pumps are operated by perfusionists during surgery. CPB is a major form of extracorporeal circulation. In modern heart-lung machines, an extracorporeal membrane oxygenation is generally used for long-term treatment.

During open-heart surgery, a heart-lung machine is an apparatus that does the work for both the heart (i.e., pumping blood) and the lungs (i.e., oxygenating the blood). The most basic function of the machine is oxygenating the venous supply of blood in the body and then pumping it back into the arterial system which helps in smooth circulation. For the body, CPB oxygenates and circulates blood mechanically while bypassing the lungs and heart in a skillful manner. To maintain perfusion to the other organs and tissues of the body, it uses a heart-lung machine while the surgeon tactfully works in a bloodless surgical field. The surgeon properly places a cannula in the right atrium, femoral vein, or vena cava to withdraw blood from the body without any additional hindrance. Venous blood is completely removed from the body by using a cannula. Finally, before returning it to the body by a mechanical pump, it is filtered, warmed or cooled, and oxygenated. The drug mixed with the blood is called Heparin and it works as an anticoagulant and makes sure that the blood that is outside the body in circulation does not get clotted. The whole process is done in a closed-loop model with utmost caution so that any air embolism does not occur, which can be fatal. Lastly, the cannula utilized to return oxygenated blood, most of the time, is inserted in the ascending aorta. But it may also be inserted in the axillary artery, femoral artery, or brachiocephalic artery.

John Gibbon and Frank F. Allbritten Jr. were the first individuals to perform a successful open-heart procedure on a human basically using the heart-lung machine. Gibbon spent more than two decades in "a lifetime of research" to develop the machine, which in technology was ahead of the times. This astounding miracle was performed on May 6, 1953 at the Thomas Jefferson University Hospital situated in Philadelphia. They skillfully repaired an atrial septal defect in an eighteen-year-old woman. In the mid-1950s, the surgical teams notably Kirklin and Richard DeWall further developed Gibbon's machine into a reliable instrument. When Barnard was at Minneapolis, he got the opportunity of being exposed to one of the first teams in the world using the heart-lung machine. This was one of the most important steps in the development of an idea of open-heart surgery in Barnard's mind and he applied it when he went back to South Africa.

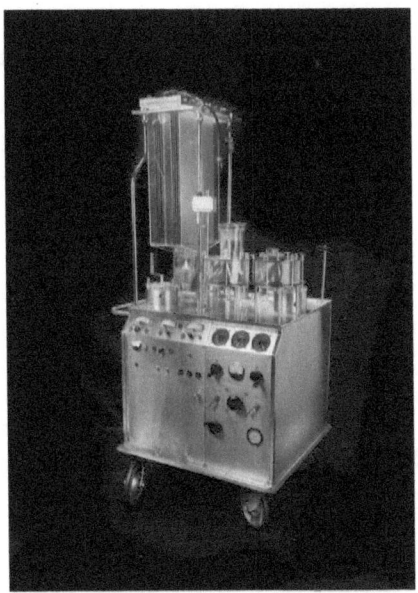

FIG: The Mayo-Gibbon heart-lung machine. It was patterned after the Gibbon heart-lung machine designed by John Gibbon, M.D. in 1949. Four years later John Kirklin and his associates at the Mayo Clinic in Rochester, Minnesota began using and improving upon a Gibbon-type heart-lung machine.

"Hypothermia technique", on the other hand, reduced metabolic need of the heart and helped in prolonging the time for surgeons to operate avoiding the toxicity of chemical build-up. The heart is a prodigious consumer of metabolic energy of all organs of the body. It is the highest consumer of energy for every gram of tissue. After the heart, the brain is also a major consumer of energy being of significant weight than all the other organs, and this is more so when the body is at rest. These two organs along with the kidneys are the things most prone to injury when the blood circulation and subsequent metabolic supply cease during the open-heart surgery.

Moreover, heart metabolism depends on the condition of the body being in rest or activity. This is because the heart rate is a significant contributor to the metabolic need of the heart. Heart rate varies from species to species. For adult humans, it ranges between "seventy and one hundred beats" averaging about eighty beats per minute. For a blue whale, which is the largest animal on the earth, it is a mere six to twelve beats per minute. **For a little hummingbird, the heart rate at active flying is an amazing 1200 beats per minute or about twenty-two per second.** That tells one more about the amazingly higher metabolic need of the hummingbird. It is true that they can be considered as the tiniest birds on the planet; nevertheless, the Ruby-throated hummingbirds are the biggest eaters among all. It has the fastest rate of metabolism amongst all the animals. At a comparative level, a hummingbird's metabolism is roughly a hundred times that of an elephant. They burn food so quickly that they often eat 1½ to three times their weight in nectar and insects per day.

For controlling mediastinal structures' bleeding that is not possible with standard CPB, hypothermic circulatory arrest (HCA) is a very useful adjunct to CPB as this allows for a bloodless operative field while smoothly maintaining cerebral protection. During the "low-blood-flow" periods of surgery, hypothermia is considered to behave as a brain protector by cooling the brain to a great extent.

The precise mechanisms by which hypothermia provides protection during myocardial ischemia-reperfusion are not well defined. One possible explanation is that hypothermia reduces metabolic demand in the myocardium at risk as a result of down-regulation of cardiac myocyte metabolism, thus helping in limiting the area of myocardium at risk. By the function of the hypothermia, myocardium is able to preserve ATP, "the basic energy currency of cells". It is a mechanism similar to the hibernation of animals in extreme cold climates. The present techniques for reduction of global myocardial ischemia during cardiac surgery with CPB include mild-to-moderate hypothermia, various types of cardioplegic solutions and different approaches for infusion of this solution into the coronary circulation.

There were two principal ways of cooling the heart during circulation. The first one is the systemic method. The idea is the blood while passing through the heart-lung machine would be cooled to the required temperature. The other process was topical or local by applying ice packs or iced water saline. Often it was a combination of both hypothermia and heart-lung machine which yielded much superior results in patients undergoing open-heart surgery. This also paved way for further difficult surgeries like heart transplant or complex cyanotic heart surgery.

While Barnard had dedicated himself to achieving a successful heart transplant, he was certainly not the only cardiac surgeon working on this. In fact, many dedicated teams of surgeons were hitting their heads on this issue even before Barnard came into the field. Among all the surgeons, the most notable was Dr. Norman Shumway from Stanford University. In the early 1950s, Shumway and his team did several groundbreaking works in the research of heart transplants. Shumway was a meticulous, brilliant yet media-shy surgeon. His team validated the technical feasibility in a dog model at Stanford University in the year 1958. This milestone in medicine was the beginning of a huge race for numerous physicians and researchers to make this operation a clinical reality.

The second team was led by Dr. Richard Lower from the Medical College of Virginia. He was previously an associate of Shumway and later established himself in the transplant research. There was also a third serious contender for the victor's wreath for the first transplant: Adrian Kantrowitz—the charismatic, unbelievably industrious, and persistent cardiac surgeon of Maimonides Hospital in New York. During those days, the scientific community quite deservedly believed that one of the three teams would make it to the title of "first successful human-to-human heart transplantation". After all, these teams were backed by the American Government that was ruling in the times of the Cold War. Facing challenges and being beaten by the Soviets in the early stage of the space race—it was the USSR that sent the first man to space—the American Government decided to significantly increase assistance to science and technology research works. Millions of dollars of assistance poured in as assistance for cardiac research from the US health department.

Barnard, on the other hand, had none of the above backing in finance, personnel or equipment. He had a bare minimum team of assistants and technicians. His nurses were the same who did routine operation as well as ward management. But he was intrigued by the idea to perform heart transplantation at Groote Schuur Hospital and therefore made it a major focus in his department in the early 1960s against all odds. On the basis of the extensive cardio-surgical experience while Shumway and coworkers were further refining the surgical technique in these years, Barnard was already convinced about the technical feasibility and wanted to enter this new field of cardiac surgery.

To accomplish his goal, Barnard knew, he had to learn more about immunosuppressive therapy and its application in transplant surgeries. He, therefore, spent a few months in Richmond, VA, USA. There he not only learned about immune suppressive therapy, which is an essential part of any transplant surgery, but he also gained a lot of firsthand knowledge about postoperative care.

In 1966, when Barnard returned from his stay in Richmond, at a major international conference Shumway and colleagues announced, "they would be ready for a first human patient." **Despite the obstacles, Barnard would beat the able American surgeons and their well-equipped teams in due time to take the pole position of the "most talked-about" surgery in the medical history.**

***

Why exactly did heart transplant become such an emotive news drawing worldwide response making it the most reported of any surgery or medical procedure of the century? The surgical procedure itself, though being challenging and innovative, was not very difficult to achieve. Many cardiac surgeries which can be imagined as much more complicated like complex cyanotic heart disease repair, neonatal switch for transposition of great arteries, or even multivalve replacement operation, to name a few, were done around the same time, but could only receive marginal public coverage. The "visceral emotion and media-hype" heart transplant achieved are unparalleled in the annals of medicine. The explanation probably lies in the ancient myths and symbolisms linked to the heart through the ages.

Heart has always been considered the repository of emotions, the anchor head of feelings. The heart has long been used as a term referring to the spiritual, emotional, moral, and in the past it was also referred to as an intellectual core of a human being. The word *heart* continues to be utilized in a spiritual sense referring to the soul or spirit, just as the physical heart was once widely believed to be and was considered as the seat of the human mind—the "stylized depictions" of hearts are extremely prevalent symbols representing love. From ancient times till now, philosophers, scientists and religious texts have tried to understand the mysterious beating structure inside the thorax—and this will continue in the future as well.

Man's curiosity and effort to understand about the heart is an ancient phenomenon. Aristotle, the great Greek philosopher, during the fourth century BC identified the heart as the major organ of the living body. According to his observations in chick embryos, the heart is the first organ to form. It was the basic seat of intelligence, sensation, and motion—this was mainly a "hot, dry organ". Aristotle carefully noted down his observations and described it as a three-chambered organ. According to him, the heart was the center of vitality in every living body. He then made a very astounding mention; his observations told him that the other organs surrounding it (e.g., the lungs and the brain) simply existed to help in cooling the heart.

Galen in his treatise, On the "Usefulness of the Parts of the Body", written during the second century AD, reaffirmed day-to-day basic ideas about the heart as the basic source of the innate heat of the body and as that organ which is most closely related to the soul: "The heart is, as it were, the hearthstone and source of the innate heat by which the animal is governed." A number of its unusual physical properties were also meticulously observed by him. As he stated, "The heart is a hard flesh, not easily injured. In hardness, tension, general strength, and resistance to injury, the fibers of the heart far surpass all others, for no other instrument performs such continuous, hard work as the heart." He boldly believed and argued that the contraction and expansion of the heart were in the true sense a behavior of its role as an intelligent organ: "The complexity of [the heart's] fibers was prepared by nature to perform a variety of functions; enlarging when it desires to attract what is useful, clasping its contents when it is time to enjoy what has been attracted, and contracting when it desires to expel residues."

William Harvey is credited with the new-age explanation of blood circulation. He supported the Aristotelian notion of the heart and its function. In the year 1653 he noted down: "The heart is situated at the fourth and fifth ribs. Therefore [it is] the principal part because [it is in] the principal place, as in the center of a circle, the middle of the necessary body." He examined all the procedures carefully and minutely observed the function of all of its different parts. At last, Harvey came to a conclusion which was reverse to what Galen and his medieval Renaissance readers believed in. According to Harvey's belief, the heart was most active at its work when it was hard, small, and contracted (*systole*), expelling blood, and then mainly at rest when it was much larger and completely filled with blood (*diastole*). In 1628, he wrote: "The heart's one role is the transmission of the blood and its propulsion, by means of the arteries, to the extremities everywhere." This observation of Harvey is one of the oldest and most accurate descriptions of heart and circulation.

Despite his scientific approach, Harvey did not challenge the metaphysical interpretation of the heart. In the late twelfth century, Master Nicolaus had aptly and rightly observed that the heart was the primary 'spiritual member' of the body. As such, it was the seat of all emotions. "If indeed from the heart alone rise anger or passion, fear, terror, and sadness; if from it alone spring shame, delight, and joy, why should I say more?" This statement was made by Andreas de Laguna in 1535. Metaphorically, Harvey brilliantly described the heart as the 'sun' or the 'king' of the body to underscore its huge cosmological importance.

When philosopher scientists tried to explain the heart in a physiological manner, the religious scholars and texts also used the heart not as a functional organ but as "a repository of faith, belief, and love". Christian scholars explain the heart as a seat of emotion and mind through scriptures. Let us note what the Bible says. According to the Bible, our 'heart' is a composition of each and every component of our soul—our mind, every emotion, and will as well as the most significant part of our spirit, which is our conscience. It is said in Matthew 9:4, "And Jesus, knowing their thoughts, said, Why are you thinking evil things in your hearts?" Here one can see that the Lord Jesus asked the scribes why they were thinking in their hearts, though it is known by all that thinking is something related to the mind. From this one can clearly understand that our mind is basically a part of our heart. When we revisit John 16:22, we find it is stated, "Therefore you also now have sorrow, but I will see you again and your heart will rejoice, and no one takes your joy away from you." We rejoice with our emotions, and here we see that our heart rejoices. As we might expect, this shows us that our emotion is part of our heart. The Lord tells us in Mark 12:30, "And you shall *love* the Lord your God from your whole *heart*." As we might expect from the religio-philosophical discourse, our intangible heart is our loving organ. **Without our heart, one could not feel the sense of love, know about love, or fall in love in return.**

The Jewish belief of the seat of the emotional and intellectual life, "Keep thy heart with all diligence; for out of it are the issues of life" (Prov. iv. 23), refers to the moral and spiritual as well as the physical life.

In Hinduism mythology, in the Ramayana, there is an episode with Lord Rama and Hanuman and there is a beautiful description in such context. After the great war was fought with the Demon King Ravana and it finally came to an end, Rama came back to Ayodhya and was crowned as the King. One day he held a court session to reward all who helped him to rescue Sita. After giving gifts and praising them, Hanuman came to visit him at the end. Rama told his nobles and ministers about the details of Hanuman's dedication and narrated to them how nobody could match Hanuman in his valor and endless service. Rama told Sita, "Hanuman's service cannot be valued." Mata Sita then rewarded Hanuman with a precious necklace that she was wearing as a gift. But Hanuman immediately refused to accept the gift as it was devoid of Lord Rama's name. People present at the court mocked him and laughed at him. They asked him to prove his love and devotion to Lord Ram. They ended up challenging him to show if Rama–Sita were residing within him or not. Hanuman stood up in front of everybody and did something unbelievable. With his own two hands, he tore his chest apart showing his heart to everyone. Everybody sitting there watched Hanuman with their mouths agape. Lord Rama and Sita were literally residing in his heart!

According to Ramana Maharshi, a Hindu philosopher, "The godly atom of the Self is to be found in the right chamber of the heart, about one finger-width's distance from the body's midline. Here lies the Heart, the dynamic Spiritual Heart. It is called *hridaya*, is located on the right side of the chest, and is clearly visible to the inner eye of an adept on the Spiritual Path. Through meditation you can learn to find the Self in the cave of this Heart."

Sri Ramana Maharshi taught that the heart, and not the head, is the true seat of consciousness; but by this he did not mean the physical organ at the left side of the human chest but the heart that beats for the right decision, and by 'consciousness' he did not mean thought but the sense of being or pure awareness of the human life. He had found this from his own experience to be the center of spiritual awareness and then found his experience confirmed in some ancient texts. When his devotees were instructed to concentrate on the heart, it was this spiritual heart on the right that was referred to; and they also found it to be the center of an actual, almost physical vibration of awareness. Moreover, he would also consider the Heart as equivalent to the Self. He would remind all his devotees repeatedly that the spiritual heart is not in the body at all, as to be specific, it is spaceless.

In the Islamic philosophy, the heart, or the *qalb*, is the main origin of intentional activities. It is the primary cause behind all the intuitive deeds of a human being's life. The *qalb* is majorly responsible for apprehending when the brain throughout handles the physical impressions. The heart and brain join forces to work together; but no matter it is always the heart where the truth or the actual knowledge can be obtained. It is important to note that the word *qalb* is used more than one hundred and thirty times in the Quran.

At that moment, it was no surprise when "the millennia of religious, scientific and deeply acculturated beliefs" of human society came to be challenged with Christiaan Barnard's work. It created a sensation; the whole scenario that the heart is an ordinary tissue which can be replaced by a few mortals standing inside an operation theater was a contra-thought and an awakening at the same time. It was like Galileo saying the earth is not the center of the universe. One might definitely get upset with him but then immediately feel a new sense of knowledge, a sense of strange empowerment, and an exciting curiosity. After all, human knowledge has always moved forward throughout different eras breaking many taboos and myths. There is just an initial resistance.

Many family members and parents of prospective transplant patients and donors refused initially to allow surgery saying that the soul of their beloved person or child remains in the heart. Many American surgeons faced the threat of being charged with homicide when they expressed their desire to take the heart of a brain-dead person that was still beating. It enraged some people when some cardiac surgeons proposed their observation without giving any emotional thought and considering the heart as a mere pump. The scientists' description of the heart as a regular 280 gram of muscle with four valves and a few pipes to control blood flow in our mortal body was too much for some people to handle.

There was a "barrage of criticism" from the media as well as the medical profession. As quoted by *The Guardian* in 1968, a consultant cardiologist working in the London Hospital described heart transplantation as "almost amounting to cannibalism." Even a cartoon was published in a British newspaper that showed cardiologists as "vultures waiting around their sick patients to snatch away the precious organs for their personal glory or profit or both!"

Barnard was also dissuaded by his colleagues and team from venturing into the unknown daring the uncertainty. Such resistance, however, deterred little or was negligible to those scientists who were determined to challenge the medical gospel. Their sole motive was to help those patients who really had within them only hope for being alive. The idea and moment of reckoning for the process of heart transplant finally dawned on humanity because of that fateful night of surgery at

Groote Schuur Hospital. To be precise, Barnard literally put "the final suture" on it.

***

Barnard rightly received worldwide recognition for his transplant surgery. He was invited by top medical universities all around the world and was requested to speak about his astounding achievement. He also gave numerous public and television appearances. He definitely had a "magnetic personality". Many governments and heads of the states would call him for advice to improve their own countries' health care. His work was recognized by the world in the form of numerous awards and recognitions that he received. He was presented with many honors, including the Dag Hammarskjold International Prize and Peace Prize, the Kennedy Foundation Award, and the Milan International Prize for Science besides being nominated for the Nobel Prize for medicine in 1968.

Dr. Barnard's surgical skill and daring behavior catapulted him almost overnight into the role of an international opinion maker. His views on almost everything from global politics to jogging to race relations were eagerly sought by the heads of the states, the United States Congress and the general public. He was no doubt a great orator and loved to speak in public. His candid viewpoints, engaging smile, and sense of humor came to the fore in media interviews. The irresistible combinations of his good looks, wits and readiness to travel and expand his reach quickened his journey to fame. He mixed with the rich and famous, developing a taste for the 'good life'.

However, with fame also came its downside. He was soon acquiring the reputation of a playboy. He would be seen more with the famous Hollywood stars and models in the most happening places rather than the operation theaters. He was soon enrolled as a member of the jet-set and became involved in a tempestuous affair with an international sex symbol. At the age of 48, he divorced his wife ending twenty-two years of relation and married the teenage daughter of a multimillionaire. But that was Barnard all along; whether professional or personal life Barnard never walked a line drawn for ordinary people by the establishment. He always chose his own path and drew his own line.

During the early 1980s, two traumatic events occurred in Barnard's life. These made an emotional impact on Barnard. His eldest son, who himself was a young Cape Town doctor, died an untimely death. Soon after his second marriage came to an abrupt end. Barnard had the problem of rheumatoid arthritis affecting his finger joints since his days at Minneapolis. Over a period it became aggravated. Barnard could do fewer surgeries than before. He retired from surgical practice in 1983, at the age of sixty-one.

Barnard afterward got involved in several business interests, including Cape Town restaurants and a cattle farm. He also involved himself in the transformation of a large sheep farm in the Karoo which later was converted into a game reserve. With the Swiss Clinique La Prairie, a profitable advisory role was also adopted by Barnard, whose primary base of interest was in the "controversial field of rejuvenation" that was done by injecting extracts from the fetuses of sheep. However, his involvement in the advertising campaign of Glycel, a cream purported to help prevent aging of the skin, somewhat tarnished his image. He continued to be active in various advisory roles, writing books and traveling for speech.

No matter whatever ups and downs he faced throughout his life, Barnard used his fame to benefit the poor and oppressed people of South Africa as they struggled under apartheid. This is because he genuinely felt great compassion for human beings of all races and nationalities. He established the "Dr. Christiaan Barnard Foundation" to provide funds for charitable and humanitarian causes. Although not openly anti-apartheid, Barnard believed in equality of all races. His patients were never discriminated against on the ground of race. Barnard exhibited an unforgettable blend of vision, intelligence, action, kindness, charm, warmth, and humor, even though tempered by human frailties. Despite everything, he successfully made the world a better place for many.

***

Barnard's work released the pent-up force of surgeons around the globe. There was a huge surge in the activities in the field of heart transplants. In just a few days after the first transplant, on December 6, 1967, Adrian Kantrowitz performed the world's "first pediatric heart transplant" at Maimonides Hospital in Brooklyn, New York. The donor infant was an anencephalic baby with a brain that was grossly malformed. The recipient infant was a nineteen-day-old baby who had the heart conditions of tricuspid atresia and Ebstein anomaly.

On January 6, 1968, Norman Shumway successfully performed the first adult heart transplant at the Stanford University Hospital in the United States. In the United Kingdom, a team led by Donald Ross performed the first heart transplant on May 3, 1968. And likewise, the era began to roll on and ventured into a bright future. Within the next couple of years, more than a hundred and forty-seven surgeries were performed all around the world.

The media and public intensely followed the development of transplant surgery at each center. More than a hundred heart transplants were performed worldwide in the year 1968 and forty-seven different medical teams participated in this medical glory. Each transplant was attended by vast publicity that crossed new lines for a traditionally reticent medical profession.

However, there was a significant problem in initial period, that went unnoticed amidst the excitement. The patients of the initial set of transplants "fared poorly" except for a few. In the New York case of transplant, the infant's new heart stopped beating after seven hours and could not be restarted. At a following press conference, Kantrowitz emphasized in a disheartened manner that he did not consider the operation a success at all. In the Shumway case, the patient died after only fourteen days of surgery.

As per Washkansky's condition, the first case of heart transplantation at Groote Schuur Hospital done by Barnard, the situation worsened after the first few days of improvement. On Day-twelve of the operation, Washkansky developed complications after staying well in the initial days and looking healthy while talking to his family amidst the media. Washkansky developed a mild fever and cough. Doctors did some tests on him and decided that the heart received by Washkansky was being rejected by his body. This was an erroneous decision and would cost the team dearly.

If a new tissue is put into a body or is placed on its surface, rejection is a normal reaction. The body's immune system reacts the moment a person goes through the process of the heart transplant. Immune cells can attack the new heart. Medicine can help to prevent this. But in many cases, rejection is inevitable. Our immune system's job is to "find and destroy things in the body that may cause harm". This includes bacteria and viruses or even any transplanted foreign body like skin graft or organs such as heart, kidney, etc. The immune system works to help keep us healthy. But in some cases, one can even be led to problems due to the immune system's response.

During a heart transplant, a surgeon basically removes one heart and replaces it with another heart from a donor. The recipient's immune system sees the new heart as a threat and can start to attack it. After a heart transplant, one needs to take medicine for the rest of his/her life. This is mainly prescribed so that rejection of the new heart can be prevented. Without regular follow-up to preempt transplant autoimmunity or missing medications might lead to rejection.

In Washkansky's case, the doctors at Cape Town Hospital increased antirejection medicines that suppress body immunity. But the unfortunate side effect was that Washkansky developed pneumonia and the situation turned from bad to worse. The antirejection drugs reduced his ability to fight germs and bacteria which affected his lungs. His lungs were inflamed and he developed severe breathlessness. He was then given antibiotics and put on respiratory support. Doctors worked round the clock to save Washkansky. In spite of the prayers hailing from every corner of South Africa as well as the world at large, he finally succumbed to death on the eighteenth day of the heart transplant. Postmortem was conducted after the unfortunate death and it showed that Washkansky's new heart was working perfectly. There were "no signs of rejection". Rather, there was an infection of his lungs. The unfortunate error happened just because the technology to diagnose and differentiate rejection from infection was not yet available in those days. In spite of a successful surgical procedure and post-op recovery, Washkansky succumbed to his regrettable death.

It was a complete heartbreak for Ann Sklar, Washkansky's wife. But it was also a big pain for Edward, Denise's father. He lamented saying that "the last part" of his beloved daughter was gone now forever. Along with Ann and Edward Darvall, the whole world seemed to mourn the death of Washkansky who was by then familiar to everybody by the daily bulletins and interviews.

Barnard was heartbroken. **"I never felt so lonely as the morning Washkansky died. For a while, I hated to get up in the morning. But I found security in turning to helping man again. For the second transplant," Barnard said in an interview.**

Barnard did not give up hope. He carried on with his research and performed surgery on other patients. Between December 1967 and November 1974, he performed ten transplant surgeries at GS Hospital in Cape Town. Barnard performed his second transplant operation on January 2, 1968. The patient was called Philip Blaiberg and he thankfully survived for nineteen months. Blaiberg's heart was donated by Clive Haupt, a twenty-four-year-old black man who suffered a stroke, inciting controversy during the time of South African apartheid, especially in the White-African press.

Blaiberg, after being discharged, walked out of the hospital on his own, went to the beach and public places, and made great media opportunities. Blaiberg's success story gave the world hope that one day heart transplantation will give sick patients what it promised in the first place. "A dream of a normal healthy life, surrounded by family and free from the dreadful pipes, oxygen cylinders and needles trapped inside isolated hospital rooms." Four lived longer than eighteen months among these ten patients, and two among these four became long-term survivors. One patient of Barnard lived for more than thirteen years and the other for more than twenty-four years.

On the contrary, the other centers were not doing well at all. Many centers, in fact, had no multi-team members and adequate facilities to achieve what was needed for a procedure of magnitude. Moreover, the volume of cases was so thinly spread that except for a few centers or its surgeons, none could scientifically follow-up or do any improvement by data analysis. Failures in heart transplants started coming up from all over the world. Examples of early death from days to weeks after surgery became common. The brief period of survival was even more aggravated by painful side effects of steroids, rejection episodes, and recurrent infections. Patients would die in a swollen-up state and were often comatose while being tethered to an array of tubes and wires. It was painful as the patients died in isolation away from their families. "It was a miserable progress of surgical science".

A total number of 107 transplants were carried out by sixty-four different surgical teams within twenty-four countries, in the year right after Barnard's surgery, that is, 1968. But it was observed that the best a patient could expect from his surgery was a span of two-year survival rate of only ten percent. By 1970, just within two years, the number of worldwide heart transplants sharply dropped from 107 to sixteen, due to the high mortality rates. In the end, even a proposal was made asking to ban heart transplants outrightly. Along with the disappointment of failure came the criticisms from media, people, ethics and religious organizations. As each case was so widely reported with a keenly interested media, "there was simply no place to hide".

The first heart transplant performed in the UK, on May 3, 1968 was done at the National Heart Hospital in London. It was performed by Donald Ross. The donor was Patrick Ryan and the recipient was 45-year-old Fred West. Patrick Ryan was a building worker and ended up suffering a terrible head injury in a workplace accident. The injury was so severe that he could not have survived at any cost. Even so, wild claims raged against the case and it was rumored that "Mr. Ryan was murdered brutally for his heart". Thus, the case went for a thorough investigation. At last, the allegation was found completely false at the inquest. After a long court case, the verdict came in their favor. But just like this incident, many such hostile receptions awaited the heart surgery pioneers.

The real problem was not in the failure of surgery or in any technical fault. It was but natural that a new procedure will have its hiccups and teething troubles. But the extraordinary media frenzy increased public expectation to a sky-high level. Moreover, too many centers jumped into cardiac transplant surgery expecting name and fame without going through the basic preparations and understandings. The result was nothing but a poor outcome and a subsequent backlash. Slowly most of the teams stopped conducting transplant surgeries. The next few years were a period of lull. Only four centers continued to do some meaningful work during this mundane period. Among them were Dr. Shumway at Stanford University Hospital and Dr. Barnard from Cape Town.

Barnard had by then been keeping away from fundamental research of heart transplant as he was being captured by his own larger-than-life image. He would be traveling around the world leaving the hospital in his younger brother's capable hands and asked him to take responsibility in the time of his absence. He could only give little time as he was busy in his extravagant lifestyle, relations, and nonclinical interests. The complete responsibility of furthering the improvement of heart transplant technique, medications and improving survival fell upon the shoulders of Dr. Shumway.

Dr. Norman Shumway was the Chief of cardiac surgery at the Stanford University. He was the doctor credited with pioneering research, groundwork, and animal experiments leading to heart transplant years before most other teams. Afterward too, when most surgeons gave up in the 1970s, he had the persistence and vision that it could work. From post hoc analysis, he knew the operative procedure was working very well. But the recipient's body was often rejecting the donor-heart. Shumway was convinced that there had to be a way to overcome transplant rejection for the long-term success of the operation. He started working on a "novel medicine" called cyclosporine, then recently discovered and used for other indications.

Cyclosporine was discovered by "sheer luck". In Sandoz, a Swiss pharmaceutical company based at Basel had asked the employees while going on business trips and holidays to take plastic bags with them for collecting soil samples. These soil samples were later cataloged and screened for any beneficial fungal species for clinical use. In March 1970 in the Microbiology Department at Sandoz, the fungus *Tolypocladium inflatum* Gams was isolated by B. Thiele from two such random soil samples. Looking like beautiful orchid flowers under scanning electron microscope this class of fungus was of a previously unknown entity to the Sandoz research team. The fungus was cultured, filtered and metabolites analyzed for any novel clinically useful molecules. This was finally experimented with and filtered to find the molecule cyclosporine.

Initially, scientists had hoped it to have antibacterial or antifungal power. To their surprise, they found cyclosporine was an immunosuppressor of human T lymphocytes cells. Since the T lymphocytes were the principal weapon against transplanted hearts in the rejection process the discovery of cyclosporine was a landmark achievement in this regard. The discovery of immunosuppression by cyclosporine in 1976 is attributed to JF Borel, a Belgian microbiologist and immunologist who was the Head of the Immunology Department at Sandoz at that time.

Cyclosporine was the strongest immunosuppressor to be discovered at the time. It also overcame many of the risk factors associated with previous antirejection medicines like azathioprine being relatively nontoxic to the bone marrow. With the introduction of cyclosporine, the patient morbidity fell. It became possible to transplant organs with a one-year success rate higher than the previous ones. The clinical trials proved that cyclosporine had an "excellent ability to suppress host immunity without causing bone marrow toxicity or other side effects". When suitably combined with other drug cocktails cyclosporine started working fairly well to prevent rejection of organs through immune mechanism.

The hearts showing early symptoms of rejections were appropriately treated with antirejection medicines with good results. Shumway worked quietly and diligently on other fronts too overcoming several technical problems. He applied himself to the careful selection of donors and recipients, made efforts to increase the donor pool, brought about improvements in organ preservation and followed developments in antirejection drugs protocols.

Another problem was to find which hearts were showing rejection and to what extent. For this, Shumway found a technique as well. He simply used a bioptome, a pincer-like device that is made to enter through neck veins and take tissue samples from the right chamber of the heart. In 1965, R.T. Bulloch initiated the concept of introducing a biopsy needle through the right external or internal jugular vein so that it could reach the right intraventricular septum of the heart and thus it could then successfully serve the purpose of sampling the heart muscle. By studying tissue cells from the heart as retrieved, pathologists could tell the stage and severity of rejection. Thereby, the impending rejection of transplanted organs could be thwarted by dose adjustment of antirejection drugs.

Armed with the abovementioned knowledge and superior postoperative clinical care, Shumway started heart transplant surgeries with new vigor. And this time, God blessed his team with success. Patients started surviving for years and decades rather than days and months. Soon the good news spread across the world and other centers also started replicating the Stanford team's success in heart transplants.

***

Cut to the modern era of cardiac science. Today, the heart transplant procedure has achieved success and acceptance as a viable therapeutic option for heart failure patients who have exhausted the other treatment modalities like medical management and reparative surgery. Regarding the long-term survival as a marker of the success of any procedure, the cardiac transplant has come a long way since the early days. In general, 85 percent to 90 percent of the patients can survive at least for one year and up to 80 percent survive for three years. A fairly good count of sixty percent of patients with terminal heart illness can hope to survive ten years or longer. With the support of advanced cardiac diagnostics and critical care that is available today, it has become a fairly successful procedure, like any other top-end surgeries conducted in big hospitals.

Along with long-term survival, most of the patients who survive the first year have an excellent quality of life. Many are able to have good outdoor life, most can go back to do office and physical work. Many also raise a family and have kids and enjoy watching them growing up. **There are hundreds of long-term success stories of heart transplants around the world. One of the notable stories is that of John McCafferty from the UK.**

In the year 1982, John McCafferty was told that he only had five years to live when he received the transplant at the age of thirty-nine. Hailing originally from Shotts in North Lanarkshire, he had been diagnosed with dilated cardiomyopathy, a disease of the heart muscle. But McCafferty went on to live another full thirty-three years after his transplant operation. World-famous cardiac surgeon Professor Sir Magdi Yacoub performed McCafferty's transplant at Harefield Hospital, west London, on 20 October of the same year. After thirty-one years, he was officially recognized as the "world's longest surviving heart transplant patient" by the Guinness World Records in 2013. He was gifted a life of more than three decades with the help of the new heart. In the end he died of sepsis and renal failure aged seventy-three at Milton Keynes Hospital. Three years before his death, he had an emotional reunion with his surgeon with Dr. Magdi. Both cut a large heart-shaped cake to celebrate the occasion along with the other staff.

"I want this world record to be an inspiration to anyone awaiting a heart transplant and to those who, like me, have been fortunate enough to have had one. My advice is always to be hopeful, to look ahead with a positive mind, and, of course, to follow the expert medical advice," John McCafferty said with pride in his eyes while he was called on stage to receive his certificate from the Guinness Book team.

Immediately after the surgery in 1982, McCafferty made a remarkable good recovery. He also ran half-marathons, took up swimming, and even participated in the well-known British and European Transplant Games. Along with his wife, he also traveled all across the world and raised a beautiful family. These are the inspiring and extraordinary success stories that motivate surgeons to remain focused on their work whenever they meet "failures or challenges."

***

In September 2001, an international news wire came which was also carried by most prominent media organizations. Dr. Christiaan N. Barnard, the South African surgeon who performed the world's first human heart transplant in 1967, died in Cyprus at the age of seventy-eight. This was tragic news for everyone across the world. Dr. Barnard, unfortunately, suffered a fatal asthma attack after going for a swim at a coastal resort in Paphos in the morning. He was visiting the place as a relaxing vacation tour. Writing the obituary, a newsman commented that "Barnard, at his death, must have been happy and satisfied knowing the surgery he did on that fateful night thirty-two years back is now a true success with thousands of cases worldwide found in all major hospitals giving new life to so many persons and their families".

Barnard, as his nature, was always hopeful and positive about the prognosis of his patients and the result of his surgeries. He would never shy away from a difficult surgery nor turn away any surgical candidate even if the odds were against him. Barnard once said in an interview in the context of his own ailment of rheumatoid arthritis, which was diagnosed during his early surgical career when he was in the USA for training, **"Always give a patient the brighter side of life. Even when conveying bad news. Because when there is hope, they will fight for life."** By the time of his death, he had already been married thrice, traveled the world, written bestseller books, and lived his life to the fullest. Indeed, he was that kind of doctor and a human being who always looked at the brighter side of life, no matter what.

***

Heart transplant brought with it many unanswered ethical, social, and religious issues. The financial burden of a single procedure to save one life when so many pressing medical problems were unattended due to poverty was criticized by many. In societies burdened with unequal living standards and private health care often not the "most deserving", but the "most affording" would go on to get that elusive chance for life. Many times, the first-world country citizens would hop over to receive a transplant from a third-world country. Organ donation (OD) processes and patients' right to privacy would also be questioned as challenged by the intrusive media.

From a noble intention, it seemed as if it would turn to "great games between players with contrasting interests and lobby."

In the selection of recipients, the characteristics of recipients such as gender, race as well as socioeconomic status should not have a primary position. A foundational paradigm grounded in justice is required by the ethical treatment of the organ transplant recipient. Justice for both the donor and the recipient ought to be the grounding principle guiding organ transplant.

Religious scholars' thoughts initially about organ donations (OD) were ambivalent. Violation of the human body after death was considered taboo by almost every important religion. However, over the years, the social thoughts and benefits of giving another suffering life a chance have found consensus. All the major religions and belief systems today broadly support the principles of OD and transplantation and accept that organ donation is an "individual choice". While live organ donations like kidney and liver are less controversial, the definition of brain-death and donation of an organ from a body have been a matter of debate in a few religions even in modern times. Everybody agrees, however, that Organ Donation is a personal matter, though being guided by socio-religious norms. Like any new concept, view or social event, the final consensus would hopefully be found in the times to come.

Some curious and many times "bizarre events" would, however, beset the post-transplant patients that has not been fully explained even today. Many of the patients would undergo significant behavioral changes after surgery. Even stranger is that some of these behaviors of recipient-patients would track and replicate the transplant donor. The recipient would many times mimic the food preference, hobbies and behavioral pattern of the donor. The dressing pattern and even love interest of the donor person would be mimicked by some recipients often to the surprise of family members. Personal habits would somehow get transferred to the recipients, and this was noticed several times.

David Waters, a heart transplant patient, acquired an "irrational craving" for a kind of snack known as Burger Rings. Surprisingly, his donor was apparently a fanatic of Burger Rings. There was another patient who hated avocados but began to relish these after receiving an organ donation. Other than food and preferences, it is also noticed that people undergoing organ transplants were seen to develop new interests, hobbies, affinities, and even new skills. One such person is Sharron

Coghlan, aged forty-five, who found that not only her tastes in food but also her interests in music, books, and movies drastically changed after an operation.

What is the reason that these people have developed these strange personality traits, quirks, and even apparent memories after receiving their organ transplants? Is there somehow, some part of the donor woven into these organs and living on in the new body, or is this something else? Several innovative ideas were put forward over the years, and many times it was even said that this is some sort of spiritual attachment. But the most accepted reason behind this phenomenon is a theory called 'cellular memory', which proposes that our blood and organs hold some essence of us, indeed even retaining hints of our very being and memories.

When a small part of ours is in form of cells, tissue, and organs, when this is transferred to another, it would allow us to live on. It will not merely be an organ but a part of our whole being. It would transfer a portion of our self—thought and behavior—along with the physical organ. "Cellular memory is the concept that memories and personality traits can be stored in any individual cells or in other organs, not just in the brain". It is just like a rose plant branch grafted on another bringing its own color of flowers and fragrance. There is some evidence for cell memory substantiated for other life forms, including flatworms and Aplysia sea slugs. But human organs are too complex and differentiated genetically to give in to such simplistic explanations.

One such documented case of a heart transplant was a story that seemed almost like "lifted from fiction". A man from Georgia received a heart transplant from a person who had shot himself. Then in the later years, he married the donor's widow. In the end he surprisingly died the same way in which the donor died. It was a self-inflicted gunshot wound. This bizarre news was reported in media in the following words:

Authorities investigating reported no foul play was suspected in 69-year-old Sonny Graham's death at his Vidalia, Ga., home. "He was found Tuesday in a utility building in his backyard with a single shotgun wound to the throat," said Greg Harvey, a special agent with the Georgia Bureau of Investigation. Graham, who was Director of the Heritage golf tournament at Sea Pines from 1979 to 1983, was on the verge of congestive heart failure in 1995 when he got a call that a heart was available in Charleston. That heart was from Terry Cottle, 33, who had shot himself, Berkeley County Coroner Glenn Rhoad said, "Grateful for his new heart, Graham began writing letters to the donor's family to thank them." In January 1997 Graham met his donor's widow, Cheryl Cottle, then 28, in Charleston. "I felt like I had known her for years," Graham told The (Hilton Head) Island Packet for a story in 2006. "I couldn't keep my eyes off her. I just stared." "After sometimes they started seeing each other. Sonny finally married the lady. Things were good for some times after which this tragic and eerily similar incident happened in which Graham shot himself with a revolver."

While very interesting, the phenomenon of 'cellular memory' is poorly understood, and there are certainly skeptics of the idea as well. The opponents of the cellular theory argue that an intense feeling of gratitude and togetherness combined with the effect of medication and anesthesia might lead to a feeling of personality change including a change in diet or outfit, which happens to be similar to the donor's because of shared knowledge of meetings with donor's family members.

It is obvious neither scientists nor the patients have been able to accept the process of heart transplantation merely as a question of "casually replacing an organ that cannot function any longer". Since the heart is often perceived as a source of love, emotion, and focus of personality traits, one must look at the situation from multidimensional viewpoints.

Only a few well-conducted studies regarding personality change after heart transplant are available in the literature by transplant psychologists. One such study was conducted in Austria, Vienna on forty-seven patients who had undergone a heart transplant. The patients were studied over a period of two years to gain insight into the problem of whether transplant patients themselves feel a "change in personality" after having received a donor-heart.

After conducting interviews, three groups of patients could be identified: 79% stated that their personality had not changed at all postoperatively. In this group, patients showed massive defense and denial reactions; they would quickly change the subject once posed with the question. It was classic signs of a massive defense and denial reaction, trying to avoid the question which can become a mental minefield if get ingrained into someone's psychology. Fifteen percent accepted that their personality had indeed changed, but not because of the donor-organ, but due to the life-threatening event. Six percent reported a distinct change of personality due to their new hearts. These incorporation fantasies forced them to change feelings and reactions and accept those of the donor. The opinions gained from interviewing these heart transplant recipients show that they seemed to be truly believing that their personalities had changed and mimicked donors to a varying extent.

How does this exactly explain distinct memories of the deceased persons returning to terribly haunt the living recipients of these organs? This is known by none. Nor could anyone figure out the real reason behind these bizarre incidents. Hence, it has somewhat become a rather "unusual and a little-explored corner of the unfathomable paranormal realm".

***

Heart transplants have caught the fascination of not only the medical community but also the media and public. Even in the modern movies, both in Hollywood and elsewhere, the fascinating story of heart transplant has been woven into many storylines simulate interesting real-life situations.

One such movie is *John Q*. It is a 2002 American drama film starring Denzel Washington and directed by Nick Cassavetes. The plot shows a happy family where the father John Quincy Archibald and the mother

Denise helplessly witness their cheerful young son Michael suddenly collapse at one of his baseball games. John is informed that Michael has an enlarged heart after a series of tests were done at the hospital. The doctor said Michael will need a heart transplant.

John was in a massive fix as his health insurance has been changed as the company he worked for suddenly dropped him from full-time to part-time, and the new policy could not cover the surgery. The only option they were left with was to raise $250,000 to get their son's name on the transplant donor list. The family tries in vain to raise the money but unfortunately is only able to acquire only a meager third of the necessary payment. The doctors are helplessly bound by the hospital rules and thus release Michael after they got tired of waiting.

Denise becomes panic-stricken and urges John to do something for their son. Unwilling to let his child die, John took up the path of crime to save him. John, in an emotional and rash decision, walks straight into the hospital ER with a menacing handgun, gathers helpless hostages, and sets strict demands. He just wanted his son's name to be on the recipient list immediately. In this chaos, Lt. Frank Grimes, the hostage negotiator, stands down to let John regain his proper senses. There is a series of tense hostage negotiation failing which John is injured by a sniper bullet. Thankfully, in the end, his innocent child is able to get the treatment that he deserved for his heart condition.

In another very successful Malayalam Indian movie named "Traffic", released in 2011 and directed by Rajesh Pillai, a different but equally interesting story unfolds. In the plot, created by award winning screenwriters duo Bobby and Sanjay, one television journalist Raihan while going for an important interview gets hit by a vehicle in a serious road traffic accident. He pitifully goes into a coma. At the same time in another city about 150 kilometers away, a rich film star's daughter, who was already a heart patient, suddenly falls ill and her condition worsens. After being persuaded by the doctors, Raihan's parents agree to a "heart donation".

Now, it is the responsibility of the city police commissioner to make the precious organ reach its destination. It is a tough journey by road as the flight is unavailable due to bad weather. The police commissioner sends an expert police car driver with the doctors by creating a "green corridor" in an exciting drive through the crowded roads. The whole drama unfolds amidst the personal turmoil and transition of the characters in the thriller simulating the adrenaline rush the real-world transplant team goes through while trying to make an organ available for surgery within the stipulated time.

In another successful Marathi movie, 'Bucket List'; the famous and talented Bollywood actress Madhuri Dixit made a comeback in her first Marathi film. In this movie, she plays very convincingly the role of a dutiful housewife who is suffering from a terminal heart condition. She is given a heart transplant which becomes successful. She then feels the urge to visit the donor girl's family—the parents and her twin brother. She comes to know of the bucket list, a wish list, the girl had prepared to accomplish before she turned twenty-one years of age. But she died tragically before that and thus her wishes were unfulfilled. Madhuri feels pity and decides to do those things, which were the fanciful dreams of a young woman such as Harley motorbike ride and playing football. While helping the girl's family in fulfilling the girl's wish, she goes to discover her own self in a beautiful way.

***

In the modern era, a heart transplant is a "multi-disciplinarian effort" in today's cardiac centers. Patients admitted in the present-day hospitals will not be having a single doctor like Dr. Christiaan Barnard to be taking care of them, even though there may be one transplant surgeon who oversees the whole program. More often, particularly in successful transplant centers, there is a whole group of experts looking after different aspects of the complex procedure. Once a patient is referred to the team, the patient is first assessed for the suitability for the transplant.

Not everyone who needs a new heart is a candidate for a heart transplant. This is because of the wide range of information needed to know if a person is "eligible for a transplant or not", a transplant team will review the evaluation. In total, the team includes a transplant surgeon, physician assistants or nurse practitioners, a transplant cardiologist, one or more transplant nurses, a psychiatrist or psychologist, and a social worker. Other team members may include a dietitian, a chaplain, a hospital administrator, and an anesthesiologist.

Basically, the transplant evaluation process must include social and psychological evaluation besides the detailed medical assessment. To be precise, the primary social and psychological issues that are involved in the process of organ transplant include extreme stress, support from family or significant others, and to top it all the financial issues. All these factors to a great extent affect how the patient responds after the transplant. After that, the person will go through an array of blood and diagnostic tests. Tests may include echocardiogram, angiogram, X-rays, ultrasound procedures, CT scan, pulmonary function tests (PFTs), and dental exams. Women may also get a Pap test, a mammogram, and a gynecology evaluation. This will help assess the overall health of the patient. Moreover, it helps in finding a good donor match and helps to improve the chances that the donor-heart, a precious commodity by any standard, will not be rejected. The prospective recipient may receive several vaccines to reduce the chances of acquiring deathly infections that can in the end affect the transplanted heart to a certain extent.

It is the transplant team's responsibility to consider all the information received from the interviews conducted according to the patient's health history, diagnostic test results, and the findings from the physical exam when deciding if somebody is eligible for a heart transplant or not. At this stage, many patients will fail to progress to the next stage that is of the transplant listing. They would be advised to continue the medical management. Some patients of high-risk category are rejected for transplant procedures and are offered ventricular assist devices (VADs) to sustain their weak hearts.

Patients who need a heart but fail to move to the list usually have some serious co-morbidities that place them at high risk for surgery or post-op result. One common cause is irreversible pulmonary hypertension or elevated pulmonary vascular resistance. When the right chamber of the heart works for long under high pressure, it develops higher blood pressure to initially cope with. But soon the lung vasculature becomes damaged irreversibly as the pulmonary system being a low-pressure system cannot tolerate such extreme pressures. Such patients, even after getting a donor-heart, would not benefit from it and will have a very brief survival span. Heart-and-lungs combined transplant may be an option for a few of them which is decided after further scrutiny.

Other causes of rejections from the candidates are active systemic infection, active malignancy or history of malignancy with a probability of recurrence, and inability to comply with the complex medical regimen. Some other times it can also be severe peripheral or cerebrovascular disease and irreversible dysfunction of another organ that may limit prognosis after heart transplantation.

Besides the causes mentioned above, there are a few other conditions that may make the prospective recipient "temporarily or partially unfit", which is either the condition can be improved upon or the transplant team after group discussion may decide that the risk involved is acceptable. In that case, the patient is enrolled. Insulin-dependent diabetes with severe organ dysfunction is one such cause. Other causes of relative contraindications of transplant are "recent thromboembolism such as stroke, severe obesity, age over 65 years, active substance abuse such as alcohol, recreational drugs, or excessive tobacco smoking".

Once a patient is accepted as a transplant candidate, he will be placed on the Organ Sharing list. The candidates are selected by an algorithm based matching process based on the severity of their condition, blood type, and body size as soon as a donor-organ becomes available. When the candidate is on the shortlist, he needs to be "on alert" to go to the hospital on very short notice, as the donor-heart has an extremely short ischemic time of only four-to-six hours.

In the United States, there is a universal listing made by the computer system for the "UNOS, the United Network for Organ Sharing", a non-profit, scientific and educational organization established by the U.S. Congress in 1984 and located in Richmond, Virginia. As mentioned earlier, patients are primarily listed according to the height, blood type, weight as well as urgency. The patients are divided on the list as per clinical status into four major categories. The categories of urgency are as follows:

1A Patients who are very sick and are admitted to the hospital. They have the equipment or mechanical devices to keep their hearts beating.

1B Patients who may be in or out of the hospital. They have intravenous (IV) medicines or a mechanical device to keep their hearts working.

Then there is Status 2 where most patients are out of the hospital and stable. And lastly, there are Status 7 Patients who are temporarily inactive on the transplant list.

In the United Kingdom, a potential patient for a heart transplant will undergo various tests and finally be labeled as "suitable, potential for future transplant or unsuitable". The suitable patient will be put on a list with the tags of age, blood group, body weight, etc. Also, an urgent or semi-urgent tagging will be done. When an organ becomes available, the recipient will be decided according to the table and match. To be on the "urgent list", it is essentially meant being in the hospital on inotropes, with a short-term mechanical circulatory support device, or even an intra-aortic balloon pump. All the other patients will remain on the "routine list". The patient listed as urgent will have the access to suitable donors from all across the UK. It was as opposed to just the local retrieval zone, for routine transplants, situated within the area of the transplant center.

With the increase in survival and awareness of the heart transplant as a treatment facility, a new issue has developed. In a paradoxical situation that can be labeled as a "crisis of success", most centers and countries have encountered a shortage of sufficient number of donor-hearts for transplant. In most western countries at any time, the number of prospective recipients on the waiting list far exceeds the suitable matched donors. There are hundreds of hospital patients waiting for a heart transplant across the world. They are completely relying on an organ donor to save their lives.

The waiting list for hearts has increased by more than 130% in the last decade. More people are being referred for heart transplants as knowledge and awareness around heart transplants have grown. Newly discovered medicines for heart failure, vaccines and antibiotics have prolonged the lifespan of end-stage heart failure patients. VADs, the mechanical assist devices are being often to support a failing heart to maintain cardiac output. The ability to use VADs also means patients can wait longer. The net result is a large number of sick heart failure patients at any point of time looking for a lucky break, a suitable donor-heart.

The average wait for an adult who needs a heart transplant is nearly three years, that is an average of 1085 days, in the National Health Service, United Kingdom. In the United States, a study showed that waiting time varies from 14 to 19 months depending on several factors. Former US Vice President, Dick Cheney, waited for twenty months after being listed for transplant and was implanted with a left VAD (LVAD). As such, these patients are hanging at a thin margin of safety after being listed for transplant. Long waits up to several years for a transplant donor to be available to be matched to the recipient means many of these patients will die before being matched. To tide over a looming crisis, cardiologists often resort to implanting VADs (Ventricular assist devices) as a substitute to a heart transplant.

Ventricular assist devices (VADs) work in various ways to support a failing heart. These are basically implantable mechanical heart pumps. A type of mechanical circulatory support device that helps pump blood from the lower chambers of the heart called ventricles to the rest of the body. Initially designed and intended for use to tide over acute crisis in persons whose heart function suddenly deteriorates, these are increasingly being utilized as a substitute for transplantation. For assisting in cardiac circulation, a VAD is most of the time used to completely or to partially replace the function of a heart that is failing. When in patients it is analyzed that the waiting time for a transplant procedure will take too long (for the size, blood type, HLA antibody status, unstable heart failure, etc.), VADs are implanted to act as a bridge to transplantation. This can now reverse end-stage heart failure so that these patients are discharged from the hospital and live relatively normal lives. VADs have been used to buy more time for patients who require undergoing heart transplants while they anxiously wait for a donor's heart.

Usually, the long-term VAD is mainly used to act as a bridge to transplant, keeping the patient alive and in a reasonably good condition, and then they are able to wait for the heart transplant by being outside the hospital. Other 'bridges' include a bridge to decision, bridge to candidacy, and bridge to recovery. In certain cases, it is noted that VADs are used as destination therapy as well. The patient, in this instance, shall not undergo heart transplantation. Moreover, the VAD is the only thing that the patient will have to use for the rest of his life. Unlike the natural heart transplanted from a donor, the VAD needs continuous maintenance, a source of power of a battery and the possibility of infection and clot formation inside the mechanical parts, making it as yet an imperfect substitute to the God-given one.

To overcome the shortage of donor-heart, many countries have enacted legislation to facilitate organ donation. Most countries have by now passed the Transplantation of Human Organs Act (THOA) in which the brain-death concept was legalized and organ procurement from heart-beating and brain-dead donors was facilitated. To be precise, an actual organ donor is basically a living or deceased person from whom at least one solid organ or some part of it could be recovered to be used for the purpose of transplantation. But in brain-death, though one is declared dead, organs are still alive and kept viable through an artificial support system. Patients classified as brain-dead can have their organs surgically removed for organ donation.

Not only legislation, the awareness by media, voluntary organization, and strong political support is often needed to support organ donation (OD). Many countries have legislated so that as a person gets a driving license, he is automatically screened for consent of OD. As in most countries, an automobile accident is the common source of healthy heart donation, and this becomes useful. It helps the bereaved family members to convince for Organ Donation as the will of the donor is already clear from his agreement or disagreement during receiving a driving license. Some countries have gone even a step to make automatic consent of all citizens who die in the hospital setting unless expressly denied by the individual beforehand. Many governments run advertising and internet promotions of the donation to make people aware and motivated. "**The US Government organ donation Unit runs a campaign saying one donor can save eight lives** (one heart, two lungs, two kidneys, one liver, one pancreas, one intestine)."

Many countries have varied rates of success in organ donation (OD). Spain has consistently recorded the highest deceased OD rate of 35.1 per million population (pmp) followed by the US (21.9), the UK (15.5), and Sweden (13.8). Although having a population of over a billion, India, like many developing countries, lags far behind in the organ donation campaign and has a national deceased donation rate of <1 pmp.

Every year, approximately 5200 heart transplantation surgeries are conducted worldwide in the present times. North America and Europe account for most of these cases. While North America which includes the United States performs about 3200 cases, Europe does 1500 cases per year. Less than 350 cases are done by the rest of the world. There is a huge disadvantage of the developing countries' citizens as far as facilities and success of cardiac transplant surgery suffering from end-stage heart failure is concerned.

India's very first heart transplant was done by Dr. Prafulla Kumar Sen, a vascular and cardiothoracic surgeon from Mumbai. Sen led the first human heart transplant procedure in India in 1968 and became the fourth surgeon in the world to carry out this operation. But the patient died within some hours of the operation, and this is mostly discounted in several scientific registries of the heart transplant list. After the Transplantation of Human Organs Bill finally received the President's assent on 7 July 1994, a group of surgeons led by P. Venugopal successfully performed India's first heart transplant at the All India Institute of Medical Sciences (AIIMS) on 3 August in the same year.

The first heart transplant in Asia was performed in 1968 by Dr. Juro Wada at Sapporo Medical University, Japan. However, the initial experience met with poor outcomes until cyclosporine was used in the year 1980. Moreover, cultural taboos surrounding organ donation (believing that OD might mean removing organs from a body before death) and incomplete legislation regarding brain-death retarded widespread heart transplant in Asia. However, the heart transplant era in Asia eventually began again in 1987 in Taiwan and Thailand, in 1992 in Korea and Hong Kong, and in 1999 in Japan. The first heart transplant in Sri Lanka was carried out in the year 2017 at Colombo in Kandy General Hospital. Thus, "the knowledge Barnard started in Cape Town has spread to all parts of the globe giving hope to sick hearts over the last fifty years".

***

Procuring and transporting a human heart for transplant is a "race against the time". Once the beating heart of a brain-dead donor is stopped and removed, its cells begin to show stress from lack of oxygen. If the time in which the donor-organ stays outside the donor body and the time before the organ is being connected to the transplanted person are longer than specified hours, the cells and structural support of the interstitial spaces degenerate. This time is called "the ischemic time". For the heart, it is barely four to six hours. This is much less than other organs like the liver and pancreas of CIT (cold ischemia time) twelve to fourteen hours and kidney of twenty-six hours.

Hearts implanted after ischemic time have the risk of acute graft rejection and failure. This span of time is not much for removing an organ, getting it to the recipient, and completing a complicated transplant surgery. Plus, not everyone is a suitable donor. Most conventional heart-donors are younger than 55, have no history of chest trauma or cardiac disease, and have a normal electrocardiogram and echocardiogram. Although in older age donors, the hearts which have stopped beating or longer ischemic time hearts are being used for transplant; and now aided by a surge of demand, this is more of an exception than the norm.

Before placing an organ in cold storage, doctors first flush the tissue with a 'preservation solution' to protect the organ from damage caused by extreme cold. At body temperature, cells pump chemicals in and out of their membranes to maintain low concentrations of sodium and high concentrations of potassium within the cells. But cells that are cold cannot pump efficiently. Chemicals leak across their membranes; and over the hours, the leaky cells swell up with excess fluid, sustaining serious damage. This damage was delayed by preservation solutions and this kept sodium and potassium levels in check. These solutions can also contain nutrients and antioxidants to sustain the cells and subdue inflammation. In combination with ice and a cooler, preservation solutions can keep organs viable for hours after the harvest.

At temperatures between 32°F and 39°F (0°C and 4°C), cell metabolism falls to about 5% of its normal rate, so tissues burn through their energy stores far more slowly and require less oxygen to sustain their activity. Because of this, cooling an organ helps delay the onset of ischemia, a condition in which tissue becomes damaged or dysfunctional due to the lack of oxygen. Keeping an organ on a cool surface like ice stretches the limited energy stores of its cells as well, preventing harmful metabolites from accumulating leading to the process of breaking down of the organ's tissues.

A new organ transportation device is under the process of evaluation through several clinical trials at the University of Minnesota and various other major heart transplant institutes stand to make more hearts available to the patients who are in need of these. This device is the TransMedics Organ Care System (OCS), often called the 'heart in a box'. The machine, not much larger than a rolling suitcase, perfuse a warm, beating donor-heart with oxygenated blood as it is being transported to the operating room. Traditionally, the heart is transferred and cooled to a lower temperature to prevent metabolism. After that, a dedicated chartered flight takes the organ to a faraway city where a potential recipient of the heart is waiting.

The device could have a 'huge impact' on the donor-organ allocation system, by keeping the heart in better condition for a longer period of time, and procurement teams can travel farther to retrieve a heart. And by monitoring the heart during transportation, the OCS allows surgeons to test a 'suboptimal' heart they otherwise would not risk using. "That would open the door for a lot of organs that potentially would be rejected by the transplant centers and that would increase the volume of the donor pool."

Often donor-heart has to crisscross the dense and chaotic intercity or intra-city traffic to reach the hospital of the recipient. Since the amount of time for an organ from the recipient to the donor is fixed by ischemic time, the only variable component is the time spent in transferring the organ from the donor hospital to the airport, airport waiting time, and the road travel time from the recipient city airport to the destination hospital. The surgical times of explant and implant are more or less non-variable give or take a few minutes depending on the surgeon's competency. The importance of "efficient and rapid transport" has been understood well in the context of a heart transplant.

To help in the process, the green corridor concept has been developed. The green corridor is a cleared-out, demarcated road route specially created for an ambulance that indulges in enabling harvested organs that are meant for transplantation procedure to reach the destined hospital sooner. Usually, such a corridor is created with help of local municipal and transport authorities and police commissionerate. It is a special corridor created so the vehicle carrying organ from the airport or another city can reach the recipient hospital without any hindrances. The idea of setting these green corridors for organ transportation refers to the corridors which are usually created in the country for the safety and security of VIP motorcades to bypass traffic on heavily choked routes. During these special times, the street signals are operated manually to avoid red signals as well as to manage the green corridors at the time of peak traffic hours.

By green corridor, the cities which would be normally excluded as a potential transplant recipient can be included in the list helping the efficient and optimal utilization of the organs. If a local recipient is not available by the previously listed organ share registry, the next potential beneficiary can be quickly notified. Coordination between various groups like donor and recipient hospitals, matching agency, transportation logistics and government workers like traffic police is as much important today for the successful conduct of heart transplant as much as is a great heart transplant surgeon.

***

When life began on the earth, the organisms were simple and a cluster of multifunctional cells. Afterward, organogenesis started in a few species. More than 500 million years ago, the very "first heart-like organ" appeared in our biological history. It has undergone many changes and adaptations during its evolution to reach the efficient and strong organ stage of today. **In a mother's womb, the heart is the first functional organ to develop and starts to beat and pump blood at about three weeks into embryogenesis.** A human heart weighs between about 280–340 grams in males and 230 to 280 grams in females and is roughly the size of a large, clenched fist. It can move 5 liters of blood in one minute and 7600 liters per day which pass through 60,000 miles of blood vessels in the human body. The average adult heart beats seventy-two times a minute; 100,000 times a day; 3,600,000 times a year; and 2.5 billion times during a lifetime without ever stopping. "It says volumes about the resilience of the heart and its will to survive".

The same resilience and tenacity were shown by cardiac surgeons like Barnard and many others while working toward their goal. They faced many adversaries, many failures on their course of action. But with each failure, their resolve to succeed became stronger. Jimmy Dean, an American TV personality, once said, "I can't change the direction of the wind. But I can adjust my sails to always reach my destination." Dr. Christiaan Barnard steered the treatment of end-stage heart failure to bring new hope to thousands of patients. **For these acts of courage and dedication, the cardiac surgeons were praised, celebrated, decorated, and awarded.** Their wonderful lives and works made cardiac surgery a dream profession like being an astronaut, Hollywood star, or nuclear physicist for the budding kids worldwide. From the beginning to the present day, the journey of discovery and miracles has continued. The noble profession of medicine and the practitioners has never faltered to give hope to the disadvantaged no matter what the condition is. The hope to live a life of dignity, to love, and be loved is the ultimate desire of every person's heart who is born on this planet. Every generation of doctors since Barnard has countless patient-success stories that have been told and passed on like folklores. One of them is of Isabella's, from famed New York-Presbyterian Hospital in the United States.

Something miraculous happened at the New York-Presbyterian Morgan Stanley Children's Hospital at Columbia University Irving Medical Center in May 2018. In an unprecedented back-to-back surgical marathon, three girls received heart transplants over a 24-hour period. That day, Isabella became a part of history as well. She was one of the lucky trio.

Her journey started in June 2015, when her mother, Kristin, saw Isabella, then 9, slumping lethargically in a chair in their Stony Point, New York home. At first, she thought it was just the weather as it was nearly 100°F outside. Time passed but Isabella failed to improve.

"She wasn't acting right or eating. Something was off," Kristin recalls. A visit to a local urgent care center suggested pneumonia. But subsequent tests at a local hospital confirmed something much worse: Isabella was experiencing heart failure, likely due to a virus. Other organs were also failing, due to her diminished heart function.

She was rushed to New York-Presbyterian/Columbia University Irving Medical Center by ambulance. The hospital is internationally known for exceptional pediatric heart-care, attracting patients from all around the world. Doctors there learned that Isabella's left ventricle—the chamber of her heart responsible for pumping oxygen-rich blood to the rest of her body—was alarmingly enlarged. Her ejection fraction (a measure of heart function) was less than 15 percent—a quarter of what it should be for a child her age. She received medication in the intensive care unit for several weeks. As her ejection fraction increased and her organs recovered, her care team determined that her heart had regained enough strength for her to return home and continue follow-up care as an outpatient in New York-Presbyterian/Columbia's Pediatric Heart Clinic.

For the next year, Isabella continued to take medication and was able to play sports. In 2017, as part of her routine follow-up care in the clinic, she began wearing a heart monitor to assess her heart function more regularly. Her doctor, Dr. Linda Addonizio—founder of New York-Presbyterian/Columbia's pediatric heart transplant program and the current Director of the Program for Pediatric Cardiomyopathy, Heart Failure and Transplantation—noticed that her heart was beating too quickly, with events of 'non-sustained tachycardia'. As a precaution, Isabella had an implantable-cardioverter-defibrillator (ICD) placed under the skin of her chest. The device would electrically restore her heart back to a normal rhythm if it pumped too rapidly.

She kept up with her monthly appointments. But Isabella's health conditions continued to decline slowly. By January 2018, she had a hard time keeping down food, her energy level and ability to do any physical activities significantly declined, and she just was not herself at all.

"I didn't like the way she looked," recalls Kristin, who called the doctors immediately. They told her to pack a bag and bring her back to the hospital, where she was admitted again to the ICU. This time she needed a more invasive procedure: implantation of an LVAD (left ventricular assist device) by the pediatric cardiac surgeon Dr. Paul Chai to pump for her ailing heart. She had the lifesaving LVAD surgery on January 11 and was listed as the highest status for a heart transplant the following day. Isabella remained in the ICU for 83 days and was then able to return home on the LVAD while waiting for her transplant.

If there was a shortage of transplants, the LVAD was her last option. But it is not meant as a lifetime treatment; LVAD is often used in patients waiting for a heart transplant. Kristin and Isabella's father, Marcos, were told it could take up to six months to receive a heart because Isabella has blood type O and could only receive a heart from someone with the blood type.

Her recovery from the LVAD surgery took its toll. "It took her a month just to get out of bed," notes Kristin. As a civil and environmental engineer whose expertise is pump design, she understood how the LVAD worked and learned how to take care of Isabella at home.

"My goal was to keep her up mentally. There was no room for negativity," adds Kristin, who would take off a total of ten months from work to care for her daughter. During a follow-up outpatient visit in May, they at last received good news: a donor-heart was available. Isabella, then twelve, was admitted to the hospital. Dr. Chai removed the LVAD and gave her a new heart on May 10, 2018.

Unlike her LVAD recovery, she bounced back quickly after the transplant: the breathing tube was removed twenty-four hours after the operation, she sat up in another twenty-four hours after that, then she walked down the hall a day later, and finally returned home just eight days after her surgery.

After some tweaking of her post-transplant medications, Isabella continues to thrive. She is finishing 8th grade, where she excels in math and science, and is excited to start high school. By all accounts, she is a normal teen. She enjoys cooking, going to the mall with friends, painting and pottery, playing piano, watching online videos to learn how-to put-on makeup, and playing with her Yorkshire terrier. She sees her doctors at NY Presbyterian monthly for checkups and tests, all of which can conveniently be done the very same day. "This smiling and active teenaged girl, Isabella, is a shining example of what a heart transplant can achieve and how it can give a meaningful and dignified life to people who would otherwise be dying".

Going back a few years in time, in 2009, it is the silver jubilee year of the first successful pediatric heart transplant operation in the world. On June 9, 1984, the surgical team from the New York-Presbyterian led by Dr. Eric Rose made history and astounded the medical world. The team successfully mustered all their experimental knowledge and gave a four-year-old JP Lovette 4th of Denver "a brand-new heart". Defying his poor medical condition which included multiple heart defects, JP lived until 2005 surprising everybody, probably including himself. After the first cases the techniques, protocols and results of pediatric heart transplants have massively improved.

Dr. Linda Addonizio, the Medical Director of the hospital's pediatric transplant team and current Director of transplant has the privilege to see the entire development since the inception. She has had an amazing journey since 1984 when she got the opportunity to help children suffering from terminal heart failure with a new and successful treatment. Linda is an incredibly hardworking doctor and people like her have kept the torch burning bright which was first lit by Dr. Christiaan Barnard years ago. Today Linda is actively involved in the celebratory moment of silver jubilee celebration at the hospital's pediatric wards welcoming and taking care of her follow-up patients of ages varying from two to thirty-five years. Linda is joined by a roomful of appreciative former patients. The day is marked to be made memorable by a photo media event hosted by the hospital to celebrate the anniversary.

As the group of patients and a few parents gathered for a snapshot in that room in the Pediatric Cardiology Department, it looked more like a happy family reunion rather than a roomful of sick children. Linda is beaming like a fairy godmother. It has been an incredible journey for her and the children surrounding her. She gently got down on her knees smiling as the photographer steadied everybody, and the wonderful moment was clicked to be admired forever. It was a proud moment and Linda's happiness knew no bounds. After all, she knows better than any person—the pleasure of making "a pure heart wholesome".

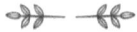

CHAPTER 3

TURN THE CLOCK BACK

"The ability to diagnose an imminent heart attack has long been considered the holy grail of cardiovascular medicine."

— Eric Topol

On the Atlantic Ocean coast of the Southeastern United States, a chain of tidal and barrier islands are mainly known as the Sea Islands. Numbering over a hundred, they are located between the mouths of the Santee and St. Johns Rivers along the coast of the US states of South Carolina, Georgia, and Florida. These are famous for their beauty and scenic surroundings. These islands are home to hotels, resorts and private beach houses, and tourists consider these as the best spot for spending their vacations.

On a Sunday, October 27, 1985, morning Andreas Gruentzig arrived at the Sea Island airport with his wife Margaret Ann. Both had spent the weekend at Sea Islands and were returning to Atlanta city where they worked. Handsome and tall, Gruentzig was already a professor of Cardiology at a rather young age of forty-six at the famous Emory University Hospital in Atlanta, Georgia. His wife Ann also worked as a radiologist at the same hospital. Gruentzig had recently purchased "his dream machine", a twin-engine private jet plane, white in color with blue strappings Beechcraft Baron. He loved to fly to Sea Islands frequently to get a breather from his hectic work schedule at the hospital.

When Gruentzig and his wife arrived at the airport, they were informed about the bad weather report warning. The meteorological conditions were unfavorable due to the occurrence of a hurricane in the Gulf of Mexico which kept getting bigger. Gruentzig, however, decided to fly back to Atlanta. The flight finally took off. The normal duration of a flight between the two locations is about two-and-half hours. But the flight never reached its destination. Soon afterward the news arrived that the plane had crashed midway with both the occupants dying in the tragic accident.

The "dreadful news" soon spread all around the world. The doctors and staff of Emory as well as many other friends of Gruentzig, practicing in several prominent hospitals in Europe and America, were deeply shocked. It was one of the saddest days for the cardiological scientific community. Dr. Gruentzig was a remarkable personality and extraordinarily famous. His invention in the field of angioplasty, the treatment of vessels of the heart and its tributaries, was discussed and praised by the world's greatest cardiac hospitals. Five years back, in the year 1980, he had been declared as "a national treasure" by the US government and was granted automatic citizenship when he arrived at Emory from Zürich, Switzerland. **By being the first person in the world to do coronary angioplasty, a novel technique to treat blockages of coronary arteries of the heart preventing heart attacks, he had created an entirely new branch of medical science known as interventional cardiology.**

Naturally, Gruentzig's death was one of the greatest losses in the world of cardiac science. An inventor, pioneer, and extraordinary surgeon's service to humanity would be untimely curtailed by the plane crash. Newspapers like the *New York Times* and television media gave glowing tribute to this heart pioneer whose inventions would go on to be the best surgical treatment ever for a heart attack. "In such a brief lifetime, Gruentzig, aged forty-six, left a "big footprint" that was difficult to fill up by anybody in the near future."

Other legends of cardiology also gave glowing tributes to Gruentzig. Spencer King, the famous cardiologist from Emory University Hospital, while speaking about him, said: "Andreas was an incredibly bright and intense guy and very committed to what he was doing, and always eager to share the knowledge. He drove fast, he lived fast, and he accomplished a lot in a short period of time."

"Andreas Gruentzig was one of the most talented, creative people on the face of the earth," said Dr. J. Willis Hurst, the famous cardiologist and Chairman of the Department of Medicine at Emory. Dr. John H. K. Vogel of Santa Barbara, California, a friend of Gruentzig's and one of the nation's leading cardiologists, said, "He was deserving of the Nobel Prize. Angioplasty is the biggest revolution in cardiology today."

The fame and adulation for Gruentzig gathered in such a brief working life was really extraordinary and worthy of praise. Why did the greatest of all American cardiologists be so effusive of the doctor from Emory who had come to the United States only recently? After all, America is not unaccustomed to medical innovations or inventions. Then what exactly was so extraordinary about Gruentzig's work? The real reason behind these emotional tributes is the dreadful history of coronary artery disease and its extraordinary influence on the twentieth century's happenings. Coming from the obscurity of the past, this cardiac disease, all of a sudden, came to being recognized and feared as the "foremost cause of death". **The great epidemic of coronary artery disease (CAD) wave began around the second decade of the twentieth century ravaging the western world and later the developing countries, in the process taking a massive toll on the young and economically active people.**

Today heart disease is the leading cause of death among people of most racial and ethnic groups in the world. It is observed that one person dies every thirty-seven seconds due to coronary artery disease (CAD) in the United States. According to CDC, the center of disease control and prevention, a US government body and leading national public health institute of the USA, it is recorded that about 647,000 Americans die from heart disease each year—that is one in every four deaths. From 2014 to 2015, heart disease ended up costing the United States about $219 billion every year. This elaborately includes the cost of medicines and health care services as well as the lost productivity due to death.

When one looks at the scenario in the UK, heart and circulatory diseases cause more than a quarter (i.e., 27%) of all deaths. This amounts to nearly 170,000 deaths each year with an average of 460 people each day or one death every three minutes. In most other countries including most developing countries the cardiac disease and mortality statistics are unfortunately on the same lines. In 2016, the estimated prevalence of cardiovascular disease (CVDs) in India was estimated to be 54.5 million. One in four deaths in India is now because of CVDs with ischemic heart disease and stroke responsible for >80% of this burden.

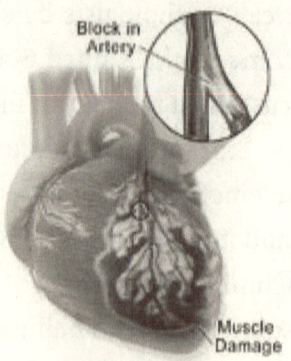

Heart Attack

FIG: Heart Attack due to Blockage of the Coronary Artery

When Gruentzig joined Medical School in Europe in the year 1958, this wave of the epidemic of coronary artery disease, which began in the first decade of the twentieth century in Europe and America, was about to peak reaching a massive scale impacting the socioeconomic milieu of these countries like no disease before or at that particular time. As a result, a huge number of economically active people with apparently normal and healthy outward appearance would fall prey to CAD. "Often this was so sudden and utterly devastating almost like a lightning, often leaving families and relatives in a state of shock".

***

Charles Frederick Hughes was a popular American football player in the Detroit Lions team. Considered as a great wide receiver in the National Football League, this young man was believed to have a bright career ahead. People were mesmerized by his charm, diligence, and skills. In an important match on October 24, 1971, the Lions hosted the Chicago Bears at the Tiger Stadium. Late in the game, with Detroit trailing 28–23, Hughes came into the field as an injury replacement.

Sometimes into the game, Landry threw a pass that tight end Charlie Sanders dropped near the end zone. Hughes, a decoy on the play, began running back to the huddle. Suddenly, things began to unravel. Out of the blue, Hughes fell on the field clutching his chest at around the 20-yard line in the stadium. His face was constricted and he was in extreme pain. While the shocked and silenced fans watched in horror, Hughes collapsed and began to convulse violently on the field.

The match-referee motioned to the sideline frantically to get Hughes assistance. Within seconds, the field was filled with the doctors and trainers from both the teams and their only focus was on trying to save Hughes. An ambulance was called for. Hughes was carried off the field on a stretcher with his limp arms dangling on the rail. The ambulance with Hughes arrived at Henry Ford Hospital, where he was pronounced dead at 5:34 pm that very afternoon. He was 28 years old.

When the postmortem reports came out, it was revealed that Hughes was suffering from "advanced and undiagnosed arteriosclerosis". One of his coronary arteries was 75% blocked and it was also revealed that he had a family history of CAD. His arteries had hardened due to atherosclerosis. He had died of rupture in one of the plaques which led to a massive heart attack.

***

Coronary heart disease grew to become a significant problem in most parts of the world by what the social medicine scientists describe as an "epidemiological transition". Initially, in a society or in a country as people are poor, they could only afford low-calorific food, due to food production being curtailed by intermittent famine or flood. Those people often die of infectious diseases like cholera, malaria, plague or tuberculosis. Other prominent reasons for death are malnutrition and hunger.

Once the people develop certain economic standards and hygiene, the cause of death changes to chronic and slow-burn diseases like cancer, diabetes, and cardiovascular causes. This epidemiological transition happens slowly over a period of decades or centuries, giving people sufficient time to change habits or make amends in food or lifestyle. In

Europe and America, right at the beginning of the twentieth century, the change was swift and unannounced by the normal standard of the medical timeline.

After a few decades, the same transition would reach the poorest nations of Asia and Africa in an even more awkward way. The situation turned from bad to worse as in these cases, the third-world population faced the brunt of modern lifestyle diseases even before coming out of the scourge of the old diseases like malaria, tuberculosis, and malnutrition. This put a double burden on the creaking health infrastructure of these pitiful countries and the disasters were much more poignant. In most cases, the disease outpaced the development of health care networks, human resources, and the infrastructure needed to manage the problem In 2001, 7.3 million deaths were recorded worldwide because of coronary artery disease. Three-fourths of global deaths due to coronary artery disease and other chronic diseases in the CAD) occurred in the low- and middle-income countries. The rapid rise in CAD burden in most of the low- and middle-income countries is attributed to multiple factors such as socioeconomic changes, increase in lifespan and acquisition of lifestyle-related risk factors developing world.

The epidemiological transition creates distinct disease patterns in various regions of the world depending on the socioeconomic stage of a specific country. The transition has been divided into four basic stages: "pestilence and famine, receding pandemics, degenerative and man-made diseases, and delayed degenerative diseases".

A dramatic shift has been noticed as the population moved through these stages and the cause of death shifted from infectious diseases and malnutrition in the first stage to CAD and cancer in most high-income countries over the last two centuries.

During the first stage of pestilence and famine, coronary artery disease (CAD) is a minor factor in the mortality table of the country.

Accounting for about 10% of deaths, the cause of cardiovascular deaths is mostly due to infection and malnutrition. Rheumatic heart disease and cardiomyopathies account for the bulk of cardiovascular death in this stage. During the second stage of epidemiological transition called receding pandemics, it was observed that per capita income and life expectancy starts to increase as the emergence of public health systems, cleaner water supplies, and improved nutrition combine completely to drive down the deaths from infectious disease as well as malnutrition. At this stage, rheumatic valvular disease, hypertension, coronary heart disease, and stroke are the predominant forms of CAD. During the next stage of degenerative and man-made diseases, the CAD comes to dominate the diseases causing fatalities. Coronary artery disease and stroke are predominant and between 35% and 65% of all deaths can be traced to CAD. In the final stage of delayed degenerative diseases, CAD and cancer remain the major causes of morbidity and mortality, with CAD accounting for 30%–40% of all deaths. The irony is, at this stage, numerous countries had achieved the status of being "industrialized, developed, or rapidly developing".

The developed countries have gone through the transitions to reach stages three or four. Most developing regions are in the early stage of transition and appear to be following a similar pattern, albeit with an alarming twist. Looking at the recent history, it is observed that the transition has occurred in the third world in a "more compressed manner". Between 1990 and 2020, coronary heart disease alone is anticipated to increase by 120% for women and 137% for men within developing countries.

However, there remain distinct differences in how severely the burden is affecting the various populations. Observing the results of various geographic regions, the rate at which CAD ranks as a cause of death is seen to vary for different areas of the world. Whereas in all the high-income countries and Latin America, Middle East as well as South Asia, CAD is seen as the commonest cause of mortality by statistics; in

East Asia, it holds the third position, and in the sub-Saharan Africa it is in the eighth place.

Even within the regions, there are many surprising variations in CAD mortality. As per the world health ranking, the highest mortality attributed to cardiovascular causes per hundred thousand population for any country is not any developed nation from America or Europe. It is Turkmenistan and Lithuania; two countries that share an astounding world's highest rate of mortality of 411 per one hundred thousand age-adjusted population. At the lowest end of the spectrum, France, Japan, and South Korea have the lowest death rate of about 40 per one hundred thousand, which is about a tenth of the rate of Turkmenistan; countries like India and the Philippines have a rate of about a hundred and forty-one per hundred thousand mortality coming about upper third of the table. A poor country like Benin or Togo has twice the death rate attributable to CAD compared to a rich country like Switzerland. There simply is not a linear relation between rich economies and heart disease as is commonly believed. The causation and effect of CAD are much more "complex and multifactorial".

***

The emergency ward of Safdarjung Hospital, one of Delhi's largest and busiest hospitals located in Ansari Nagar and perched strategically on the arterial ring road, is always a crowded place at any time of the day. It was my first posting in my Postgraduate Medicine Training as a First-Year Resident at the ER section of the hospital. As it was meant to be, the First-Year Residents like us are the workhorses doing everything from putting arterial lines, intubations, Ryle's tubes to doing minor stitches in wounds. The job is supervised by the Senior Residents who have completed their training of three years and are experienced enough having gone through all the rotations of medicines like nephrology, cardiology, and hematology.

On that evening, I checked up on the roster and found Dr. Ajay Gupta's name on the Senior Resident list. I was happy as I knew Ajay was not only experienced and knowledgeable, but he was also very friendly and easy-going telling stories from the previous postings. For a tough twelve-hour shift when you get hardly twenty minutes for food and an hour of rest if you are lucky, a senior partner like Ajay is as good as it gets.

As soon as I entered the emergency, I got busy with several cases that needed utmost attention—a severe case of poisoning, a case of acute gastroenteritis, and another case of acute nosebleed. Putting up blood transfusion and Ryles tubes and filling up proper case history notes took up a lot of time. And before I knew, three hours had passed by.

Suddenly, I got a call from the sister asking me to attend to a new patient. As I glanced at him, I saw that he was a lean-built thirty-year-old man. He did not look very sick. This is a common scenario when patients often jump to night emergency to get treatment just to avoid the long queues in the morning Outpatient Department. However, one cannot turn away any patient without a workup. I checked his blood pressure and pulse and did an auscultation of his chest. It all looked fine. Then I properly went through the entry card to read his details—Prabhat Kumar, thirty years old, male.

"What is the problem?" I asked him.

"I had a bout of sweating and sinking feeling while coming back from office in Dhaula Kuan," he said. "It happened about two hours back," he added.

Then I asked him for any past history of illness and any drug or alcohol addiction. He replied that there was none. I ordered an ECG. It took thirty minutes and the technician finally came with the ECG report. It was normal. I was not sure what to do next.

Hence, I called in Dr. Ajay and elaborated on the problem. He was also unsure about the diagnosis. However, he ordered a drip of saline to be given to be perfectly sure. In between his blood sugar was checked too. All the while, Prabhat rested on his bed and smiled amiably. He felt well now, as he said. After observing him for a good four hours and detecting no further symptoms, Dr. Ajay decided to let him go home and asked him to come back to OPD for a follow-up the very next day. Usually, the beds in the emergency, in almost all hospitals, are scarce with a huge number of serious cases streaming in any minute through the doors. It is like a war for us with twelve hours of continuous work, almost all the time standing straight without getting a chance to sit down for more than a few minutes.

Hardly an hour had passed by, when I saw Prabhat entering from the emergency door again. By this time, I had become like his friend, spending a good amount of time through the evening. I asked him what happened. Prabhat described his problem in detail. As soon as he got out of the hospital, he walked up to the bus stop on the ring road adjoining the hospital. He wanted to board a DTC bus called Mudrika to reach his home at the opposite end of the city. Soon enough the bus arrived. But the moment he settled down on the seat and purchased a ticket, the same "sinking feeling occurred again, making him feel like fainting". He stopped the bus immediately and came back to the emergency ward.

I consulted Dr. Ajay again. Both of us again went through the system-wise examination and thoroughly checked Prabhat's chest, abdomen, and conducted a neurological examination. Again the exam ended with a negative result. However, we decided to admit him this time for a follow-up scan and evaluation the next day. Since his echocardiogram and ECG both were normal, the Cardiology Resident, a pricey person always, refused to take the transfer of the patient.

This was a busy evening. There were several serious emergency cases, and I stabilized the patients with blood transfusion, analgesics, etc. After that, I had a case of meningitis needing a spinal fluid tap. Another messy alcoholic was found lying unconscious on the roadside and was brought in by the police patrol. The man was drenched in dirt, vomit, and blood. It was not clear he was unconscious due to excessive alcohol intake or head injury.

As soon as I finished attending him, one nursing staff came running from the other end calling my name repeatedly. I rushed with her to the emergency ward beds on the other side. By then Dr. Ajay had also arrived. As we observed keenly, Prabhat lay motionless on his bed, his eyes rolled up. Three of us immediately conducted a resuscitation process on him for a good forty minutes with the aid of a defibrillation, mainly adding all medications soda bicarb, adrenaline and calcium. But to no effect! Prabhat was declared dead. As I finally moved away, I guiltily looked back again. Prabhat's eyes were open as if still trying to talk to me.

What was the cause of death? Was it a myocardial infarction? With a normal ECG, it could well be an aortic dissection or a ruptured aneurysm. Or could it be an intermittent bout of ventricular arrhythmia storm leading to fibrillation or arrest? As a first-year Medicine Resident, it was my early brush with sudden cardiac death, which I continued to learn afterward and understood how unforgiving it can be. Prabhat's death remained with me as an unsolved mystery and a painful memory.

***

Richard Bruce 'Dick' Cheney served in the Nixon White House as a staffer before serving eight years as Vice President during the George W. Bush administration. Dick also served as the Chief of Staff in the Ford administration. After a series of important contributions to the Republican Party in the year 1978, Cheney was finally elected to the House of Representatives, serving five terms and becoming house minority whip.

The near-constant campaigning and Washington deal-brokering was full of challenge and stress. Cheney came up with the most common way of dealing with his hectic schedule and stress; he simply went on smoking cigarettes. Then in 1978, he had his first heart attack at the age of thirty-seven.

Cheney tried to make some lifestyle changes but ended up not following them altogether. He began smoking again, did not get enough exercise, and put on weight. The addiction got so worse that he approximately smoked three packs of cigarettes every day for almost twenty years. Then the heart attacks came as a repetition. The second one came when he was forty-three. The third when he was forty-seven. Finally, the fourth occurred just a few weeks after the crucial 2000 US presidential election when Cheney participated as running mate to George W Bush. Cheney has had five heart attacks in total, his fifth occurred in early 2010. The former Vice President thus had to go through a series of heart procedures. He underwent four vessel coronary artery bypass grafting in 1988, coronary artery stenting in November 2000, urgent coronary balloon angioplasty in March 2001, and the implantation of a cardioverter-defibrillator in June 2001.

CNN host Larry King too had a life in which he bravely fought with heart disease while carrying on with his high-pressure job as a journalist, television and radio host. At the tender age of nine, Larry had to see his father's tragic death due to a heart attack; he was aged forty-three at that time. The sudden death of his father had a terrible impact on Larry and slowly he lost interest in academics. After he graduated from high school, he decided that he would work to support his mother and never went to college. However, from very early on, his lifelong dream was to have a career in the radio business.

With hard work and dedication, Larry King achieved phenomenal success in his opted field of work. His life, however, took an unfortunate turn when, in 1987, King got his first heart attack at the age of fifty-three. Later that year, the deteriorating state of King's heart necessitated quintuple-bypass heart surgery.

Remembering his first heart attack, King had said that he did "everything wrong" prior to his heart attack. What exactly did he do? It was then revealed that in addition to smoking almost sixty cigarettes per day, King had a poor diet, experienced high stress levels due to his busy work schedule, and skipped exercise regularly.

But after his heart attack, King vowed to change himself entirely. He quit smoking, began walking regularly for exercise, and adopted a healthier diet. He was strict with his determination and cut back his intake of sodium, meat, alcohol, and other cholesterol-raising foods. King successfully thwarted his inherited bad genes with these efforts and overcame all the poor habits of initial years of life. He was able to continue his strict routine for a long period to maintain a successful career and eventful personal life.

Most people whether famous and popular people like Chuck Hughes or ordinary people from everyday life become aware of the cardiac ailments inside them only after some symptoms have occurred. They would awaken to the problem only after getting symptoms like a chest pain leading to heart stroke or loss of consciousness leading to low blood pressure or pulse. But by the time these symptoms are investigated by the doctors, often it is found that the underlying disease process of atherosclerosis inside the coronary arteries has progressed since much earlier, many times even decades. **CAD and atherosclerosis are indeed deceptively silent, often mysteriously fatal disease progressing inside the millimeter size arteries called coronary arteries running on the surface of the heart.**

The coronary artery wall is made of three layers of tissue. The outer layer called adventia is a fibrous tough layer to give strength, while the mid-layer is made of muscular cells. It is the inner layer called intima which is the most important for causation of CAD. Under the microscope, intima looks like a pavement-floor made of flattened smooth cells. For many years, it was considered as an inert layer of surface in contact with blood. But now it is understood to be much more, it is a cell bed of vibrant activity exchanging metabolites, releasing hormones, and even thinking for the heart. Depending on the physical situation of the person, intima cells decide the proper time of dilating or narrowing down the arteries, thereby adjusting blood flow to the myocardium. The intima takes these decisions autonomously by its own neural network. This is called "autoregulatory action". It is surprising to note that these complex activities do not come to the level of the conscious brain. Hence, at any moment, a person is unaware of hundreds of vital activities going on inside these tiny coronary vessels which supply blood and nutrients to the heart muscles.

The disease process of coronary artery disease (CAD), known as atherosclerosis, often begins innocuously as a small injury to the intimal layer that may result in a tear. It is frequently observed that harmful changes in endothelium may occur due to certain molecules like oxidized particles. Diabetes and a high level of cholesterol cause a change in blood flow and rheology alteration. External activities like smoking and stress can frequently cause spasm of the coronary arteries, which do not respond to a normal autoregulatory function. Hence, it is understood that all the above may lead to a minor breach on the surface of endothelium. Many unwanted molecules and degenerative particles enter through this breach and settle down in the subendothelial space. This nidus ends up further attracting harmful cells and particles like cholesterol crystals.

With the passage of time, the small nidus grows further to a large bulging structure into the lumen of the coronary artery. This is called "atherosclerosis plaque". This process often takes many years to evolve. By the fourth or fifth decade of life, the bulge has narrowed the coronary artery to a critical level in which any activity would lead to cardiac muscles being starved of proper blood flow. This causes symptoms which are clinically called angina—chest pain of cardiac origin.

"This natural history of gradual progression of atherosclerosis, however, may take an unfortunate abrupt turn in some people". The smooth endothelium and plaque may get torn apart by a sudden unexpected force. This cut on the surface of the internal lining of coronary artery, though small to the naked eye, is huge at the microscopic level. This immediately gets plugged by platelets, fibrins, and red blood cells.

This ball of tissue is called a thrombus. This is the region from where a heart attack originates.

The sudden occlusion of blood flow to the coronary artery due to the thrombus can be quite dangerous. The electro-metabolic changes unleashed by the sudden cessation of blood flow to the heart often precipitate dangerous arrhythmias. The heart beats erratically at a rate two or three times the natural heart rate. In others, the arrhythmia makes the heart to beat so chaotically that the heart simply ceases to beat gradually and end up quivering like a "bag of worms". In both situations, the result is the same—the person collapses and dies within minutes if not given urgent medical attention. **Every year hundreds of thousands of people in the world die of sudden cardiac death which most often is caused by this small seemingly innocuous thrombus of a few millimeters in size.** This is exactly what happened to Chuck Hughes on the football field at Tiger Stadium in Detroit in front of a crowd of forty-five thousand sitting in the stadium with mouths agape in horror.

***

But the above understanding of coronary artery disease is only a recent phenomenon. From "early history till mid-part of the twentieth century", the etiology and pathogenesis of CAD were vague and barely explained. There was only an anecdotal mention of the problem over the centuries by various scholars, philosophers, or historians. Just that doctors did not understand atherosclerosis accurately till the mid-part of the twentieth century, does not make it a disease of modern society. From the archeological and historical analysis, it is now well understood that CAD always existed in humans even before the millennia.

It is interesting to note that deaths with all the characteristics of CAD were described quite elaborately by the Egyptian papyruses, mortuary inscriptions, and tomb reliefs as early as 3000 BC. When certain mummies were found without any injury or evidence of common diseases of the time, it made scientists curious about what led to the death of the subjects. They began to conduct thorough research to solve the mystery behind these deaths. In the end, they came up with the hypothesis that CAD may be the cause of death particularly in the mummies of aristocratic Egyptian society who were habituated with a sedentary lifestyle and rich foods. The exact cause could only be proved by opening the heart which was difficult given the preciousness of the mummies from the high society of ancient Egypt.

CT (computed tomography) scan—a twentieth-century technology—enabled investigators to see the coronaries of the mummies without performing a dissection. An article published in The Lancet in the year 2013 describes with whole-body CT scans of mummies from four different geographical regions (ancient Egypt, ancient Peru, Ancestral Puebloan of Southwest, and the Unangan of the Aleutian Islands). The scan reports showed that atherosclerosis may be a very ancient happening. The time period spanned more than 4000 years ago. The investigators found probable or definite atherosclerosis in 34% of the 137 mummies studied. Surprisingly, one among the three mummies with coronary heart disease was the renowned Princess Ahmose-Meryet-Amon, who resided in Thebes during the years 1580 to 1530 BC. She died in her forties; it was observed that two of her three main coronary arteries were blocked. If she were a resident of the present world, she would have been instructed for bypass surgery by the doctors. From these facts, it is obvious that this disease was not uncommon in premodern humans. Early agriculture era after the settlement of colonies could be the time when the atherosclerosis process became prevalent worldwide.

Though ancient in origin, the study of coronary artery disease (CAD) was not taken up in a systematic manner for many centuries after its discovery. It was, however, William Heberden who brought angina pectoris to the attention of the medical profession when he presented his paper, 'Some Account of a Disorder of the Breast', at the Royal College of Physicians in London in 1768. In a classic description of angina, Heberden wrote, "Those who are afflicted with it are seized, while they are walking, and more particularly when they walk soon after eating, with a painful and most disagreeable sensation in the breast, which seems as if it would take their life away, if it were to increase or to continue: The moment they stand still, all this uneasiness vanishes."

The term 'angina pectoris' was first coined by Heberden from the Greek word *ankhonē* meaning 'strangling' and the Latin word *pectoris* meaning 'chest'. No matter how many years have passed with a somewhat inaccuracy in locational description, the modern era of medicine still uses this historical term 'angina pectoris'.

For more than one hundred years after Heberden's lecture, clinicians and pathologists alike were preoccupied with 'fatty change and fibroid degeneration of the heart', totally ignorant of the myocardial necrosis secondary to obstructive CAD. However, in the year 1880, Carl Weigert broke the spell and clearly described the condition of myocardial infarction, correlating the disease of the coronary arteries with myocardial changes. He recognized the etiological role of coronary atherosclerosis and the different effects of myocardial ischemia which occurs because of the reduction of coronary blood flow. If the ischemia is gradual, it causes fibrosis; abrupt ischemia may lead to necrosis of heart muscles. Soon postmortem diagnoses of coronary artery thrombosis were conducted. Finally, in 1912, James Bryan Herrick demonstrated electrocardiographic changes and brought the condition in front of the whole world.

In the year 1812, an article 'Remarks on Angina Pectoris', written by John Warren, M.D., appeared in the very first issue of *The New England Journal of Medicine and Surgery*. The description was as follows:

"The remarkable facts, that the paroxysm, or indeed the disease itself, is excited more especially upon walking up a hill, and after a meal; that thus excited, it is accompanied with a sensation, which threatens instant death if the motion is persisted in; and, that on stopping, the distress immediately abates, or altogether subsides; have formed a constituent part of the character of Angina Pectoris."

This was written about two hundred years from the present day. But Warren's description of angina pectoris is so accurate and elaborate that it is still taught to the medical students of the modern era. What is so interesting is Warren wrote it during an era when the pathogenesis of CAD was unknown. The treatments in those days consisted of bloodletting, a tincture of opium, bed-rest, or a combination thereof.

In 1856, Rudolf Virchow gave a proper definition of the physiological elements in thrombus, which is basically a blood clot within the vascular system and the risk factors that predispose arteries and veins to thrombus formation. In his studies, Virchow mainly mentioned the three factors: "stasis of blood, endothelial injury, and hypercoagulability" as the basic pathophysiology of thrombus formation. Virchow's concepts on thrombosis remained relevant to the current understanding of cardiology and the process of a heart attack. Only after Virchow postulated the features of thrombosis—the formation of a clot in the arteries and veins—did scientists begin to consider the clinical implications of coronary heart disease seriously.

Near the end of the 19th century, cardiovascular physiologists noted that experimental occlusion of a coronary artery in the dog caused 'quivering' of the ventricle which was rapidly fatal. Pathologist Ludvig Hektoen in the year 1879 came up with a conclusion that the cause behind myocardial infarction is coronary thrombosis "secondary to sclerotic changes in the coronaries." The first decade of the twentieth century was a turnaround time for the diagnosis and epidemiology of CAD. In 1910, two Russian clinicians described five patients with the clinical picture of acute myocardial infarction (AMI), which was confirmed during postmortem examination. At last, a definitive clarity was found on the causation and presentation of coronary artery disease.

***

Mark Twain, the celebrated American writer, known for his brilliant works like *The Adventures of Tom Sawyer* and *Adventures of Huckleberry Finn* faced a tragic death due to a heart attack on April 21, 1910. He was a humorist finding fun in every moment of life. It is documented that once he commented on a rumor of his death as, "The reports of my death are greatly exaggerated."

Some miraculous things were noticed during this great soul's death. When Mark Twain was about to leave this earth, Halley's Comet was passing across the skies shining brightly. One will be surprised to know that Halley's Comet was also seen near the earth on his birth year. Twain had himself predicted the event in 1909 saying, "I came in with Halley's Comet in 1835. It is coming again next year, and I expect to go out with it. It will be the greatest disappointment of my life if I don't go out with Halley's Comet. The Almighty has said, no doubt: "Now here are these two unaccountable freaks; they came in together, they must go out together." True to the words, Mark Twain's soul left his body just a day after the beautiful comet reached its closest approach to earth.

On reading about Twain's life, one will find that he himself admitted that his stage comedy performances during his youth were extremely stressful for him. Hence, he became habituated to alcohol intake and heavy smoking. Ever self-deprecating and jovial, he would sometimes say about his attempt to quit smoking, "Giving up smoking is easy… I've done it hundreds of times."

Although Twain is always celebrated and remembered for his wit and humor, his life was not smooth and easy. He suffered a series of business losses in his later life due to misjudged investments. Then after a few more years, Twain faced a major setback in life when his closest family and acquaintances left him forever. His wife Olivia's death in 1904 and daughter Jean's on December 24, 1909, deepened his gloom leaving him shattered to pieces. On May 20, 1909, his close friend Henry Rogers died suddenly. At this very moment, Twain succumbed to a deep depression. Thus, depression was also added to his list along with stress and smoking, all of which are known today as risk factors of CAD.

After losing "almost everything in life", Twain went on a tour perhaps hoping to escape from the painful memories; he traveled to Bermuda. By early April, he began having severe chest pains. His biographer Albert Bigelow Paine joined him, and together they returned back home. Finally, Twain died on April 21, 1910, presumably because of a final heart attack.

Even after the fact that the increase in heart disease, particularly atherosclerosis causing CAD, got noticed and documented in the first decade of the early twentieth century, the doctors could only do precious little regarding the treatment, such as in the case of Mark Twain. The principal reason why an understanding of CAD was so feeble amongst pathologists and physicians of the nineteenth century and earlier was that the disease itself was a mere curiosity. It may look surprising today but the prevalence of CAD up to the first decade of the twentieth century was very less and certainly insignificant compared to infectious and diseases of newly industrialized like the deadly tuberculosis.

Before epidemiological studies and death records became a regular feature, the appreciation of the importance and growing prevalence of the Coronary Artery Disease could only be noted by various small but dependable data. The coroner's court for the Liberty of Ripon and Kirkby Malzeard in Yorkshire, UK is a case one can consider as an example. From 1855 to 1926, it gives an authentic review of all the deaths, and again the deaths taking place in the period between 1981 and 1983. The records are extremely detailed in the documentation and give an accurate picture of the growing incidence and prevalence of CAD and myocardial infarction. It showed that the number of deaths from acute CAD was very low during the Victorian times but suddenly increased within the period of 1906 to 1910. It reached the peak level from 1981 to 1983. But throughout, the population of the area remained stable and was around 22,000.

Similarly, the number of postmortems for myocardial infarctions carried out in the London hospitals also provided evidence of the fact that CAD as a cause of death was much less when compared with the percentage of total deaths caused by other diseases. The study of autopsies in the city of London showed that the increase in the number of deaths from CAD began in the year 1909 or 1910. But it greatly increased between 1917 and 1923. In recent times, it is seen that every third death in the most developed countries and a few developing countries is related to heart or vascular in origin. Swept over by this "marauding killer", we take for granted that heart and blood pressure-related diseases have been the commonest cause of death always. But this is farthest from the truth as can be. **In fact, apart from the present century, the twentieth century is the only one in human history when heart and vascular diseases were the commonest cause of death.**

Throughout human history, various diseases have stood out as the most dreaded conditions often striking down hundreds or thousands of people in swift outbreaks. Since the time of the early humans, when the hunters, gatherers, and nomads settled down forming clusters of villages and which later developed into cities, the microbes like bacteria and viruses have been the major cause of several fatalities, taking advantage of close living which spread infections. If taken together, one will find that malaria was the number-one killer of all times followed by tuberculosis and smallpox. Plague, influenza, and cholera also lead the dishonor list of being the biggest killers of human history. In the first decade of the twentieth century, this pattern of infectious diseases causing deaths took a break after three thousand years of civilizations.

A decline in infectious diseases, subsequent to increased hygiene antibiotics and vaccines, initiated the change. Combined to it were the diet, lifestyle change, and longevity. Eventually heart attack and other vascular diseases came out from shadow to grab the top spot, which they have not forsaken ever since. In 1900, pneumonia was the leading cause of death in the United States, and the average life expectancy was only forty-seven. But it is seen that doctors and scientists mainly focused on treating infectious diseases during the first half of the twentieth century—for example, virtually eradicating tuberculosis as well as developing new drugs for curing pneumonia. There was a dramatic decline in the number of people dying from infectious diseases in the twentieth century. Moreover, poliomyelitis (polio), diphtheria, tetanus, whooping cough, measles, mumps, and rubella were all virtually wiped out during the second half of the twentieth century, right after the introduction of childhood immunization. These dramatic advances increased longevity and inadvertently opened the door to coronary heart disease.

The large majority of today's cardiac deaths are due to coronary heart disease that is secondary to coronary atherosclerosis. In 2009, coronary artery disease accounted for 64% of all cardiac deaths. A number of explanations are offered elaborately discussing the massive increase in coronary heart disease deaths from 1900 to the 1960s. The marked increase in deaths attributed to heart disease, from 1900 until the late 1960s, was almost certainly due to an increase in the incidence of coronary atherosclerosis, with resultant coronary heart disease. The scenario saw a transformation as people were living longer as there was a decrease in deaths from infectious diseases. But on the other hand, changes in diet led to the consumption of processed foods, more saturated fats, added sugars, and other high glycemic index carbohydrates.

One of the most noteworthy changes was the spectacular increase in cigarette smoking among the general population. Early in the twentieth century, several events coincided which contributed to increases in annual per capita consumption of cigarettes. This included the introduction of blends and curing processes allowing tobacco inhalation, improvements in mass production, the invention of the safety match, transportation permitting widespread distribution of cigarettes, and last but not least use of mass media advertising for promoting cigarettes. During the 1920s, social changes and targeted industry marketing reflecting the liberalization of women's behavior and roles led to the increasing acceptability of smoking among women; soon cigarette smoking began to increase among women. An increase was observed in the annual per capita cigarette consumption from fifty-four cigarettes in the year 1900 to 4345 cigarettes in the year 1963. This can be considered "a hundredfold increase".

Another notable aspect of contributory factor which also began during the first decade of the twentieth century was the availability of automobiles. It was not a coincidence that the number of CAD patients increased during the same period when the massive increase in automobile production and usage happened in the USA and Europe. Another twist in the event was noticed when cars entered mass production in the early twentieth century. In 1908, the Ford Model T began production and came into the market. It was the creation of the Ford Motor Company and would grab the title of being the first-ever vehicle to be mass-produced on a moving assembly line. It was also recorded that Ford produced more than 15,000,000 Model T automobiles from 1913 to 1927.

In the year 1907, the United States produced 45,000 cars. But in 1935, that is, twenty-eight years later, the number had increased almost ninety-fold to 3,971,000. The impact of such exponential rise of automobiles did have a crucial influence on various social aspects such as sedentary lifestyle, reduced physical activity, and dining out habits triggering the fast-food culture.

One more reason behind the rapid spread of CAD and atherosclerosis through the twentieth century all over Europe and the USA was the waves of urbanization. A vast number of people migrated to cities from rural agricultural communities. The nineteenth century, specifically in the period between 1820 and 1914, elaborately tells about a turning point between a society that was still essentially rural and an urbanized, developed society prefiguring the end of the twentieth century—a society within which more than 90% of the population would not be involved in agriculture anymore, though some of these might still be dwelling in the countryside.

From the beginning, an equilibrium existed between the vast majority of the population who were involved in subsistence agriculture within a rural context and small clusters of populations in the towns where economic activity mainly consisted of trade at markets and manufactures on a small scale. This broad pattern of population scatter was maintained from the development of the earliest cities in Mesopotamia and Egypt until the eighteenth century. The ratio of rural to urban population remained at a constant equilibrium due to the relatively stagnant and primitive state of agriculture throughout this period.

This rural-urban balance of population finally came to an end with the onset of the British industrial and agricultural revolution in the latter part of the eighteenth century. This was followed by an unprecedented growth in the urban population over the course of the nineteenth century. It is also observed that both of these continued through migration from all over the countryside as well as due to the extreme demographic expansion occurring at that time.

When the scenarios in England and Wales were recorded, it was found that the proportion of the population dwelling in cities consisting of over twenty thousand people showed a sharp jump from 17% in 1801 to 54% in 1891. When a wider perspective of urbanization is adopted, it can be said that the urbanized population in England and Wales, in 1891, represented 72% of the total. But for other countries, the figure was 37% in France, 41% in Prussia, and 28% in the United States.

The urbanization of the United States took a long span of time to occur, with the nation attaining urban-majority status only between 1910 and 1920. By the first decade of the twentieth century, most of the developed world of the recent times had set themselves up for urban sedentary lifestyle, which can be noted as a major precursor of the rapid increase in the prevalence of CAD. Currently, over four-fifths of the US population resides in urban areas, a percentage that is still increasing today. In Japan, the figure is 91%, and the global average of urban population is 56%.

With the rapid growth of this specific urbanization, the process of atherosclerosis hastened; and as a result, this increased the prevalence of CAD vastly. This fact is proven by several studies that compare the incidence of coronary artery disease in a few isolated tribes in recent times who still managed to keep themselves away from any contact with the modern human societies. These unique tribes continue to maintain the lifestyle of our ancestors, to be precise that of hunters and gatherers, which was basically the hallmark of ancient premodern humans.

One such study is published in *The Lancet* in 2017 and it was about a cross-sectional cohort study on the Bolivian Tsimané tribes. The Tsimané live in the Bolivian Amazon and have a pre-industrial, subsistence lifestyle of hunting, gathering, fishing, and farming. The tribe was subjected to the study to look into the heart health and risk factors at the population level. **A cardiac CT scan study was done and Tsimané tribes were found to have the world's lowest prevalence of CAD of any population ever documented.** An astonishingly low level of only 3% of the studied individuals was found to have a significant atherosclerotic disease, which can be claimed as the lowest in the world for any society that was yet studied. This happened despite having a high infectious inflammatory burden of malaria and worm infestation which is known to act as a stimulus for atherosclerosis.

The Tsimané population also had very low levels of LDL cholesterol, thus rarely having the presence of cardiovascular risk factors, such as obesity, hypertension, or high levels of sugar in the blood. The average Tsimané adult heart has a physiology of a twenty-year-old American! A Tsimané develops any risk of heart disease twenty-four years later compared to the time an American does. "It may be said that these Amazonian tribes have the world's healthiest hearts." The low levels of CAD in this forager–horticulturalist population suggest that urbanization and elimination of a subsistence lifestyle might be important risk factors for CAD.

***

While the epidemic of coronary artery disease (CAD) progressed in the first half of the twentieth century, a few seminal developments around World War II radically changed our perception of CAD and its management. With a renowned individual's death during the war-time, the people awakened to a new knowledge. When the world witnessed the US President's death, a sudden awakening of the danger CAD was aroused within the hearts of the people all across the modern globe.

Franklin Delano Roosevelt, serving as the President of the United States of America from 1933 to 1945, was in a way part of the epidemic, suffering severely from heart failure due to undiagnosed as well as untreated risk factors. He suffered from "acute uncontrolled hypertension and cardiomegaly". He suffered from headache and fatigue, even as his blood pressure was at an alarmingly upper range. Unfortunately, he almost never received any proper treatment to cure him.

On March 27, 1944, while the planning for the Allied landing at Normandy was on the verge of completion, the President got admitted to Bethesda Naval Hospital. He was suffering from dyspnea on exertion, diaphoresis, and abdominal distension. During those days, there were only a few hundreds of cardiac specialists in the entire nation. One among them was Cardiologist Dr. Howard G. Bruenn, who dutifully attended to the President. According to Dr. Bruenn's observation, the patient appeared 'slightly cyanotic' with blood pressure 186/108 mmHg. The patient's chest X-ray showed an "increase in size of the cardiac shadow." The young and talented cardiologist gave the President his very first diagnosis of "hypertension, hypertensive heart disease, and cardiac failure." The doctor preferred treating Mr. Roosevelt with digitalis and salt reduction; to be precise, this was the only primitive treatment of heart failure available in that particular era.

Just two months before his death in the year 1945, Roosevelt could attend the Yalta Conference along with Churchill and Soviet Premier Joseph Stalin; they were supposed to negotiate about the anticipated post-war administration of Germany as well as an expected future United Nations. Churchill's personal physician, Lord Charles Moran, noted down something very important in his diary, "The President appears a very sick man. He has all the symptoms of hardening of the arteries." From then, just after a few weeks, President Roosevelt bid the world his very last goodbye on April 12, 1945; he was aged sixty-three at the time. The cause of his death was a cerebral hemorrhage and his blood pressure measured 300/190 mmHg. He had succumbed to the national epidemic of cardiovascular disease in a very similar manner of numerous other Americans.

Roosevelt's death shook the people far and wide and an alert switch was pressed about the dangers of CVD. People became seriously aware of this terrifying disease. On June 16, 1948, President Harry Truman signed into law the 'National Heart Act'. It was reported, "The law allocated a $500,000 seed grant for a twenty-year epidemiological heart study, and also established the National Heart Institute, which today is known as the National Heart, Lung and Blood Institute."

At the very beginning, the National Heart Institute, later renamed the National Heart, Lung, and Blood Institute (NHLBI), established the Framingham Heart Study in 1948 and this was their first act. This basically involved the devoted collaboration of professionals hailing from three disciplines: clinical cardiology, epidemiology, and biostatistics. Their main aim was to gather knowledge about the characteristics of the human heart and to understand the formation of heart disease by elaborately studying the lifestyles of the residents of Framingham, Massachusetts. The first description of their findings was "Factors of Risk in the Development of Coronary Heart Disease," and it indicated that increasing blood pressure and cholesterol levels along with smoking were associated with an increased frequency of ischemic heart disease and acute myocardial infarction. **The study also came to the conclusion that there is a high incidence of myocardial infarction among women,** and this often appeared later in life than in the case of men. It was discovered that the female hormones had an apparent protective effect on the formation of CAD, but this was removed after the menopause span began leading to the late formation of atherosclerosis.

The identification of raised blood pressure and cholesterol levels as risk factors and the institution by the NHLBI of national programs to thoroughly educate clinicians and the public at large about the significance of controlling these hazardous factors have contributed to a dramatic improvement in the age-adjusted cardiac death rates. With the identification of these dangerous coronary risk aspects as well as the others that followed, the underlying mechanisms in angina and myocardial infarction came out into the light, thus introducing the concept that there is a chance of preventing coronary heart disease and its complications. It was subsequently revealed by the increasingly large multicenter clinical trials that both primary and secondary preventions were possible when measures were adopted to lower blood pressure and total serum cholesterol. **"The veil that masked the underlying mechanisms in CAD, angina and myocardial infarction was finally being lifted".**

Second major advancements were achieved in the field of lipids. The "lipid hypothesis", also commonly known as cholesterol hypothesis is a medical concept theorizing a connection between blood cholesterol levels and the occurrence of atherosclerotic cardiac disease. A number of trials on lipids in individuals in their sixties and showed that "measures used to lower the plasma lipids in patients with hyperlipidemia will lead to reductions in new events of coronary heart disease." In the earlier parts of 1913, Russian scientist Nikolay Nikolaevich Anichkov began to feed a diet ultra-rich in cholesterol to the rabbits in his lab. After a few weeks, he killed the rabbits to autopsy the major artery aorta and iliac arteries. Anichkov's research revealed that these rabbits fed on cholesterol developed lesions in their arteries, whereas the rabbits with normal foods did not. This was very much similar to atherosclerosis occurring in human coronary arteries, thus suggesting a role for cholesterol in atherogenesis. Anichkov postulated that the so-called "fatty flecks of arteries" are the early lesions of atherosclerosis. It was also noted by him that these may later develop into something drastic or the more advanced lesions of the disease. By the year 1951, it was accepted that fat deposition was a major feature of the disease process though the causes of atheroma were still unknown.

As Coronary Artery Disease became a common risk factor of death in the western world during the middle of the twentieth century, the lipid hypothesis simultaneously received higher attention. In the year 1940, Ancel Keys, a researcher at the University of Minnesota, postulated that the supposed epidemic of heart attacks mainly found in the middle-aged American men was heavily connected with their mode of life as well as the possibly modifiable physical characteristics. During the middle of the 1950s, Keys recruited collaborating researchers with improved methods and design within seven nations to mount the very first cross-cultural comparison of heart attack risk. It was basically designed to study the male cohorts engaged in traditional occupations in cultures contrasting in diet, especially in the proportion of fat calories of various compositions.

In the starting phase of 1957, Keys and his colleagues started with some observations which eventually would be called "the Seven Countries Study". The subjects included 12,000 men aged between forty and fifty-nine and hailed from eighteen areas of the seven countries—Italy, Yugoslavia, the Greek Islands, the Netherlands, Japan, Finland, and the United States. The communities in the study were mainly chosen for their contrasting dietary routine as well as the relative uniformity of their rural laboring populations.

Keys and his peers were able to conclude through central chemical analysis of the foods consumed by families selected randomly as well as diet-recall measures that in societies where animal fat was a major component of every meal—especially in the US and Finland—both blood cholesterol levels and heart-attack-death rates were at the peak. On the other hand, blood cholesterol was much lower and heart attacks were rarer in cultures where diets were based on fresh fruit and vegetables, pasta, bread, and plenty of olive oil—mainly in the Mediterranean region. A 1970 report clearly mentioned that dietary saturated fat can lead to CVD, and this relationship is mainly mediated through serum cholesterol. **"This ultimately had a decisive impact on CVD and**

public health prevention methods that we see today including food labeling on all packaged as well as processed foods available in the supermarkets."

Yet another simple observation in the hospitals helped in finding out a significant method for treating heart attacks. Until 1961, patients with a heart attack who were able to make it to a hospital were assigned beds located randomly throughout the hospital. They were kept far away from the nurses' stations so that their complete rest would have no hindrance. It often happened that patients were found dead in their beds the next morning, presumably due to a fatal tachyarrhythmia. Indeed, the risk of death occurring in the hospital during those days was as high as 30% compared to the present rate of 4-6%.

The first concept of the coronary care unit (CCU) was designed by Dr. Desmond Julian. With his insight into the prognosis of patients suffering from heart attacks, Dr. Julian arrived at the conclusion that the survival rates would increase if the heart patients, the proper equipment, and the efficient staff who knew how to use the equipment were present in the same place. Julian's observation led to the development of the coronary care units that provided continuous monitoring of the electrocardiogram, external defibrillation, and closed-chest cardiac resuscitation.

Dr. Julian began his career in the United Kingdom. Years later he went to work in Australia and successfully set up the world's first Cardiac Care Unit in Sydney in the year 1961. Soon he returned to his homeland in the United Kingdom thereby successfully setting up Europe's first Cardiac Care Unit in Edinburgh three years later in 1964. Hence the concept of CCU was born. Soon it became a standard feature in all the tertiary care hospitals. The Edinburgh CCU unit saved the lives of an extra seven out of every hundred patients in its first year; this seemed quite advanced compared to the old method. "The result was surprising"; it was observed that this reduced in-hospital mortality by half among patients admitted with AMI. The concept of the Cardiac

Care Unit (CCU) was thus successful in reducing mortality similar to the introduction of the seat belts in cars even without adding "any extra medicines or novel surgeries".

***

While these advancements were taking place in the preventive aspects of cardiac care, some newer surgical procedures were introduced to improve coronary artery disease treatment. After the development of cardiac catheterization, finally, nonselective angiogram became possible in the 1950s. By this technique, the coronary arteries—the obstruction of which caused heart attacks and CAD—could be fully delineated and mapped for the disease. As soon as proper data were collected, the cardiac surgeons immediately prepared proper diagnosis and advice for a treatment plan.

The discovery of the heart-lung machine was a great step in the post-war era of medical research. With the help of this machine, the heart could be stopped for a while to conduct surgery on the heart with relative ease in a bloodless field. Originally, the heart-lung machine developed by Gibbon was introduced into cardiac surgery for repairing the congenital intra-cardiac defects. But soon the cardiac surgeons adopted this for adult coronary revascularizations, popularly known as the Bypass surgery. Several techniques were devised by the surgeons to get over those stubborn blockages in the form of atherosclerotic plaques deep within the coronary arteries resulting in a deficit of myocardial circulation.

In the 1950s, the introduction of surgical coronary endarterectomy was made, which is the stripping of the intimal layer with atherosclerosis. In the coronary endarterectomy procedure, the coronary arteries were cut open and the plaques were removed. However, this did not end up becoming a standard treatment as 'intimal stripping' often led to many complications. The arteries that were stripped would often close abruptly, and this led to massive myocardial infarction and death. In 1958, the Swedish surgeon Åke Senning further refined this specific technique, by utilization of venous patches to seal coronary arteries after the removal of coronary plaques by the process of endarterectomy. After a few years, it occurred to surgeons that instead of cutting the plaque it would be easier to "bypass the blockage" by using another artery or vein.

On April 4, 1962, David Sabiston performed the first clinical case of a direct hand-sewn coronary anastomosis, during the time of anastomosing the saphenous vein graft (SVG) to the right coronary artery (RCA) at Johns Hopkins Hospital. Technically this procedure was usually performed off-pump by using an end-to-end distal anastomosis. However, the scenario took an unfortunate turn and the patient died three days later due to a sudden stroke. Sabiston became so disheartened by this experience that he did not attempt any other vein bypass for almost a decade. He even preferred not to report this important event until the year 1974. Therefore, the Russian surgeon Vasilii Ivanovich Kolesov was given attributes in the historical records for the first successful hand-sewn anastomosis. He, on February 25, 1964, completed a suture of the RITA to the RCA without cardiopulmonary bypass. And in the year 1967, he properly reported the outcomes of his first twelve bypass surgeries.

In May 1967, Argentine heart surgeon René Gerónimo Favaloro achieved a physiologic approach in the surgical management of CAD at Cleveland Clinic USA—the bypass grafting procedure. In this new technique, he used veins from the legs to replace a stenotic segment of the right coronary artery, and this was called saphenous vein autograft. As the leg venous circulation has multiple channels, removing one for using on the heart would not harm the legs at all. In the later years of his career, he successfully as well as skillfully used the saphenous vein as a bypassing channel. Moreover, this technique has favorably become the present standard bypass graft technique. In 1968, three talented doctors—Charles Bailey, Teruo Hirose, and George Green—used the internal mammary artery instead of opting for the saphenous vein for the grafting procedure.

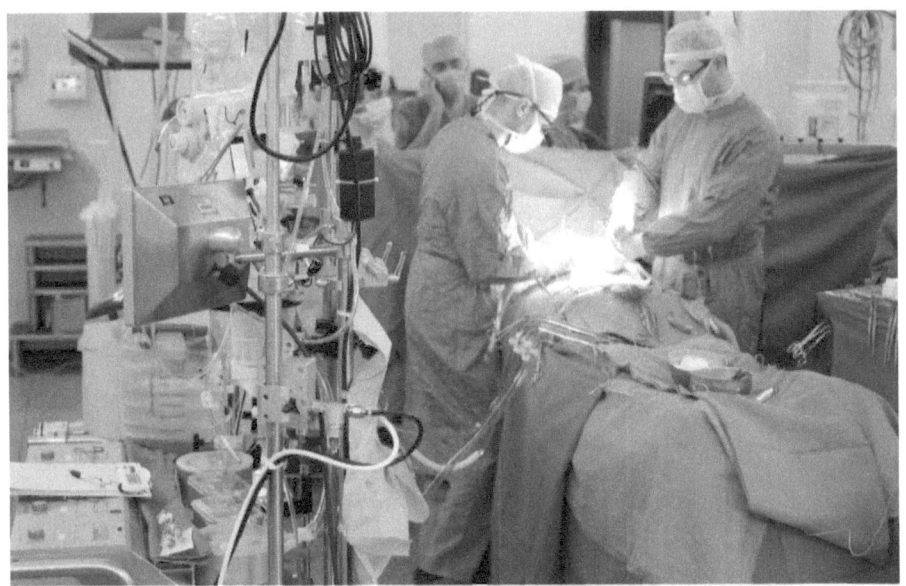

FIG: A modern heart surgery in progress with the assistance of a heart-lung machine

When coronary artery bypass procedure (CABG) became useful for the treatment of CAD, a large number of patients benefited from this procedure. But the difficulty with CABG was the use of complicated techniques which involved sternotomy by cutting open breastbone to approach heart, ventilation and use of heart-lung machine with its own attendant risk. Interestingly, other vascular beds of the human body such as femoral artery in the leg or iliac arteries of the abdomen and pelvis, blockages similar to coronary arteries were treated with an entirely different approach. The arteries of legs and hands commonly called "the peripheral arteries" were also subject to a similar process of atherosclerosis as that in the case of the heart. The resultant blockages often caused severe pain on walking or raising arms by progressive narrowing, and this is basically a sign of ischemia due to reduced blood circulation. This pain is particularly known as "claudication pain". The pain would progress to ulcer of legs or gangrene if not attended at an early stage finally leading to limb loss by amputation.

In an entirely new approach, which starkly differed from the traditional surgery, these peripheral arteries were neither dissected nor were bypassed by a surgery. The idea was no doubt revolutionary, but refreshingly simple like any other great proposal. The peripheral arteries were approached from within by a catheter inserted with the help of a tiny hole on the skin made proximally. In this manner, the blockages could be corrected by a tiny incision on the surface of the limb, instead of dissecting the skin and muscles to approach the deep-seated arteries for performing a bypass on the arteries of the leg and hands. This new technique was named "angioplasty" or moulding of the arteries, and was pioneered by two renowned doctors of that era—Dr. Charles Dotter and Dr. Thomas Fogarty.

Charles Theodore Dotter joined Medical School at Cornell and completed his internship at the United States Naval Hospital in New York State. His residency training was at the New York Hospital. At the age of thirty-two, Dotter, became the chief of the radiology department at Oregon State University in Portland. Surprisingly, his discovery of angioplasty to open an obstructed leg vessel in 1963 was an "accidental discovery". While using an abdominal aortography to assess a renal artery stenosis, he introduced a catheter via the femoral artery in the groin. Later he observed that he had involuntarily recanalized an occluded right iliac artery just at the moment of passing the catheter. He observed at the time of the removal of the catheter that the channel inadvertently created remained open, and this observation was followed with demonstrated improvement in leg perfusion. Hence, Charles Dotter believed that he could treat those vessels without surgery in view of this experience.

Thereafter, Dotter performed the first planned transluminal angioplasty on January 16, 1964 on an eighty-two-year-old female patient named Laura Shaw. Laura was severely suffering from a left leg ulcer with gangrenous toes. She was in acute pain, so the surgeons had advised amputation of the leg, but she steadfastly refused the proposal. Thus, the general surgeon referred the sick woman to Dotter.

When Dotter examined her as well as her angiogram report, he understood that she had a short segment tight stenosis of the left leg on the superficial femoral artery. Dotter used a co-axial catheter system, consisting of a tapered eight to twelve Fr Teflon catheter to progressively dilate the stenotic area. In this technique, the catheter was initially crossed across the blockage over a guidewire. Next, it was progressively upgraded to higher and higher caliber catheters exchanged over the wire to achieve the dilatation.

Thankfully, Laura's procedure went well. It resulted in the overall warming of the leg as well as the progressive disappearance of the pain with reduced stenosis. Within two weeks, the foot ulcer got healed completely. At three weeks, Dotter did an angiography to confirm the patency of the femoral artery. Laura Shaw, the first patient going through angioplasty, died three years later from congestive heart failure. But until then, she was able to walk on her two feet without difficulty. Charles Dotter discovered that atheromatous plaque on the vessel walls could be compressed like snow. This became known as 'the Dotter effect'. His method of opening up an arterial obstruction without using scalpels was named Dotter's technique.

While Dotter was treating arterial blockages with the atheromatous plaques, Dr. Thomas Fogarty on the other hand was dealing with blood clots inside the arteries called "an embolus". These clots often come into vascular flow either by local injury to the arteries or from a faraway source such as a damaged heart valve. It was observed that these clots when of sufficiently large size cause sudden acute cessation of blood flow to the limbs causing gangrene leading to amputation. "Fogarty invented the embolectomy catheter revolutionizing the treatment of blood clots of embolus".

Fogarty was born on February 25 in the year 1934 in Cincinnati, Ohio. He was brought up by his mother alone as his father died when he was eight years old. Fogarty was "a tinkerer" since childhood. He loved working on repairing things to help his mother out. He would also make model airplanes for his school friends and concentrated on working on automotive parts in his spare time.

During Fogarty's initial years while working at Good Samaritan Hospital, he witnessed the regrettable deaths of several patients who died from complications in blood clot surgeries in their limbs. Seeing about 50% of patients dying helplessly with the traditional treatment method, he was determined to find a better way for curing them. In the traditional method, surgeons had to use forceps to remove blood clots, just after a huge part of an artery had been dissected, leaving the patient under general anesthesia for hours. Since there was interruption of the blood flow during the procedures, it often increased the risk that the patient might end up losing a limb.

Fogarty's attic at his modest home was his usual place for his gadget making. One day while sitting alone in his attic, Fogarty pondered upon different ways for making the procedure better. He was very much concerned about avoiding the long and frequently risky incisions to cut open the leg vessels. He began to work on a urethral catheter and balloon. The urethral catheter used to help passing urine was similar to the size of the femoral artery. It was also flexible yet strong enough to be pushed through the blood clots forming inside the artery. He concluded that the catheter would be able to reach to the clot without much trauma to the patient as it only needed a small keyhole incision.

For creating a balloon, Fogarty mainly cut off the tip of the pinky finger of a size 5 surgical latex glove and then attempted to incorporate it onto the end of the catheter. He inflated thus creating a balloon with saline using a syringe. It was then retracted as soon as it had expanded to the size of the artery, withdrawing the clot through the artery and out of the incision. Fogarty continued improving and modifying until he got a proper usable model of balloon and catheter, which he could finally try on actual patients. Fortunately, this was found to be extremely useful. Hence, the more modified and improved version named "Fogarty's embolectomy catheter" has been used throughout the world since then saving millions of patients from leg amputations.

Combining Dotter's balloon catheter and Fogarty's clot-buster could well be the final objective for treating a heart attack, which is basically is a combination of stenosis of the coronary artery and the clot formed therein. But there were loads of difficulties on the path to success. It would thus demand a "massive amount of technical modification as well as translational medicine application" for finally achieving favorable outcomes.

While searching for solutions for curing coronary artery disease (CAD), Dotter did think that his technique may be used to relieve blockages in coronary arteries by utilizing some form of a catheter. This is because the catheter may expand the atheroma from the inside, which would have a similar effect as a bypass from outside. Hence, this would obviate the requirement of open-heart surgery and even opening of the chest in a major surgery. But this radical idea was much easier said than achieved. The potential complications were numerous; the tiny coronary arteries were 3–4 mm in diameter compared to leg arteries which have a measurement of 7–8 mm. There was the risky possibility of "rupture of the arteries" while expanding from inside. While performing a heart operation, such an occurrence would bring about a catastrophe called "the tamponade". It is also observed that this blood leak can immediately bring about the patient's death.

Moreover, the plaques may return through a recoil after dilatation, in turn making the procedure redundant. Coronary arteries were not only very slim, but also the arteries were mostly functionally "end arteries". That is, each artery was the sole supplier of blood to a particular portion of the myocardium. That coronary circulation if suddenly stopped by an abrupt closure of coronary artery by balloon catheter use could cause the death of the patient unless immediately opened by open-heart surgery with opening the chest. Several other issues including the requirement for such ultra-slim hardware effective in coronary arteries had also remained unsolved.

Before trying any experiments on the human heart, all the problems needed to be extensively experimented in canine models in a proper laboratory. As there were just too many imponderables to handle, Dotter could not pursue this idea any further. **Finally, it was the brilliant and tenacious mind of a young doctor from Germany who diligently worked upon the idea and was determined to see if it works. His name was Andreas Gruentzig.**

***

Andreas Gruentzig was born on June 25, 1939, in Dresden, Germany, just a while before the beginning of World War II. His father Dr. Willmar Gruentzig was a chemist and his mother, Charlotte was a teacher at a local school. Shortly after his birth, Gruentzig's family relocated to Rochlitz, a small historical town situated in between Dresden, Leipzig, and Chemnitz. Gruentzig's father served as a meteorologist during the war; unfortunately, he went missing just before the closing of the war and was never found afterward.

Post-war, Gruentzig's mother Charlotte Gruentzig constantly insisted that an excellent education was of utmost priority for her children. Andreas Gruentzig and his brother Johannes were admitted in high school at the Thomasschule zu Leipzig, which was considered one of the best schools of the time in Germany. In 1957, Andreas Gruentzig graduated from this school with the highest honors scores. In 1958, strongly desiring to become a physician, Gruentzig escaped from his homeland just before the Communist Government closed East Germany's borders. Gruentzig ended up joining his brother Johannes at the University of Heidelberg.

Gruentzig completed his graduation from the University of Heidelberg on April 8, 1964. After completion of his internship by the end of September 1966, Gruentzig returned to his alma mater. By then he had made a plan of pursuing a career in public health. Gruentzig's mentor, former physiologist Hans Schäfer, had become Director of the newly established Institute of Social and Occupational Medicine at the University of Heidelberg. Schäfer secured Gruentzig a postdoctoral research fellowship. Gruentzig was expected to receive a part of his training in public health and statistics in London as per the requirement of the scholarship. Gruentzig reached London to work under Walter Holland, at St. Thomas Hospital Medical School, which is presently part of King's College London.

Gruentzig also got the chance of working with Donald Reid at the Department of Medical Statistics and Epidemiology of the London School of Hygiene and Tropical Medicine. Thereafter, he completed his course in clinical epidemiology from this institute. It is noted that Reid very much focused on atherosclerosis and CAD prevention in his research. This in turn inspired Gruentzig to a great extent and helped in forming a robust foundation for his future work. It was this London training that brought about the initial impetus for Gruentzig in cardiovascular medicine. While being trained for public health, Gruentzig became particularly interested in the field of atherosclerosis and desired to gain knowledge of the same.

***

Long before Gruentzig would start his quest to solve the coronary artery problem endovascularly in the least invasive manner, many cardiovascular scientists had applied themselves to the heart and vascular diseases in previous decades. In the beginning, the foremost issue for the doctors was "how to access the inner chambers of the heart in a living person without compromising on safety."

During the 1920s, the knowledge for safe access to the heart was not known and was not possible in any manner. But it was a crucial initial step so that any pressure recording of vitals of cardiac chambers could be handled meaningfully. It was also not possible to deliver any drug directly to the heart without such an access. "The idea, however, was considered way too dangerous" at that time by almost all medical experts. It was strongly believed that any fiddling into the pumping heart from outside might either cause traumatic rupture of chambers of heart or precipitation of arrhythmias—an erratic rhythm-less contraction of the heart ending in a sudden cardiac arrest.

None could discover "the heart's inner secrets" without a safe and reliable access into the cardiac chambers. The first person to achieve success in this unthinkable task was Forssmann. **In 1929, he literally unlocked the access to the inner sanctum of the heart's chambers to be studied by the scientists.** Not to mention, the method was "utmost dramatic involving an almost suicidal effort".

Werner Theodor Otto Forssmann was born in Berlin on August 29, 1904. After completing his schooling in 1922, Forssmann went to the University of Berlin to pursue a career in medicine, after passing his State Examination in 1929. For his clinical training, he opted for the University Medical Clinic and was working under Professor Georg Klemperer. He then studied anatomy under Professor Rudolph Fick. In 1929, he went to the August Victoria Home at Eberswalde near Berlin to complete his clinical instruction in surgery.

Forssmann's "unbelievable inspiration' for performing what is now widely known as cardiac catheterization basically hailed from a nineteenth-century sketch done in his physiology textbook which depicted a long, thin tube that was to be positioned into a horse's jugular vein and guided into the animal's heart with balloon-assisted measurements of intra-cardiac pressures. Forssmann strongly believed that he too could reach the human heart but through a different access altogether. He used the veins in the crease of the arm, to be precise "the brachial veins" which are more accessible. Forssmann believed that there would be many benefits if a catheter could be inserted directly into the heart. Such a catheter could be used for direct delivery of drugs into the heart, injecting radiopaque dyes for taking cardiac images or measuring blood pressure of the cardiac chambers.

But Forssman knew on his own he could not let the experiment happen. Hence, he elicited the help of Gerda Ditzen, who was working as a surgical nurse at Auguste Viktoria Hospital, Eberswalde, near Berlin. By pursuing relentlessly Forssmann finally could convince her to become his "first human guinea pig". Forssmann sought Ditzen's help as she was the one who held the keys to the closet, which was required to obtain a long enough catheter. At last, Ditzen agreed, but Forssmann had something else in his "secret plans" she would know only later.

One afternoon while there were few people in the hospital, Forssmann took Ditzen with him inside the operating room. As soon as she was strapped to the surgical table waiting for the catheter to be inserted in her arm, Dr. Forssmann gallantly walked the distance of the OR and started his self-experimentation. Forssmann put a clean incision on his own left elbow crease. Next, he identified the predominant vein and gradually inserted a 65-cm-long ureteral tube into his arm. He had previously selected this catheter which was the only tube appropriate to the size to safely and adequately reach the endocardium. It was later revealed that at the moment Forssmann felt a painless warmth as the tube coursed along toward the heart. Forssmann carefully concealed the tube hanging out of his arm.

Then he requested Ditzen to accompany him to the X-ray room. By that time Ditzen was able to understand the doctor's crazy plan and was apprehensive, but Forssmann somehow managed to pacify her. With the tube dangling menacingly from Forssmann's hand, both entered into the fluoroscopic X-ray facility in the hospital basement. The X-ray revealed that the tube was placed in the right auricle inside the heart. Forssmann finally obtained the proof that he needed as soon as the technician took out the snap of the picture. Forssmann uneventfully removed the tube.

If we venture through history, we will come across numerous "self-experimentations" in medical science as this procedure is quite common. It has been seen that medical researchers often prefer using the newly discovered drugs, procedure or some strange gadgets on themselves as nobody was ready for the risk of trying the thing. The doctors might also be governed with the noble intention of not hurting others but self in case the new experiment did not go as it was planned. **However, all self-experimentation would pale in front of what Forssmann did that day. Perhaps his "youth and naivety" won the day for medical science as any experienced doctor would not have dared to put a urinal catheter into the heart.** In the late summer of 1929, as a surgical resident only one year out of Medical School, Forssmann performed the world's first right heart catheterization on himself. He was aged only twenty-five at that time.

Forssmann later repeated this cardiac catheterization in a septic patient in critical condition. He believed that the therapeutic advantage of directly injecting cardiac medications suprarenin (adrenaline) and strophanthin (a digitalis preparation) into the central circulation underscored the therapeutic value of the procedure. He had the intention of doing several such experiments on the field of cardiac catheterization, but he was presented with a path studded with "thorns of disbelief and blatant rejection".

"It is surprising that no immediate rewards were awarded to Forssmann though being an early pioneer of one of the most crucial experiments". Rather, his career went downhill progressively for a long time. He was facing the wrath of the conservative medical community for whom strict and mundane routine habits of medical procedures were more important than any experiments. Although initially very annoyed, the head clinician at Eberswalde finally recognized Werner's discovery when he was shown the X-rays. He decided to allow Forssmann to carry out another catheterization.

The patient chosen by Forssmann for his next attempt at cardiac catheterisation was a terminally ill woman whose condition improved to a certain extent after being treated and given drugs in this manner. After being treated as an outcast and helplessly hanging on for a job, an unpaid position was created for Forssmann at the Berliner Charité Hospital, working under Ferdinand Sauerbruch. However, Forssmann's this job also saw an abrupt end. Sauerbruch was annoyed that Forssmann had continued doing catheterizations without his approval. While dismissing Forssmann from the job, Sauerbruch sarcastically commented, "You certainly can't begin surgery in that manner."

After facing such disciplinary action for self-experimentation, he had to leave the Charité. He was re-instated again but was soon forced to leave again in 1932 for not meeting scientific expectations. Forssmann joined another hospital for a while before leaving in 1933 after he got married to Dr. Elsbet Engel, a specialist in urology in that hospital. By this time, Forssmann had been tagged as one who conducts "dangerous experiments on patients", which is not at all a suitable name for somebody hoping to make a living out of medical practice. When he failed to get a job with his reputation, he finally quit cardiology and took up urology; an unfortunate loss to the field of cardiac science research. At the beginning of World War II, he took up the position of a medical officer. During the war, Forssmann was once captured and put into a US Prisoner Of War camp. He worked as a lumberjack when he was released in 1945. Then he became a country medic in the Black Forest with Elsbet. In 1950, he resumed practicing urology in Bad Kreuznach, a small provincial town of southwest Germany.

While Forssmann was being imprisoned, his research article on cardiac catheterization was read by André Frédéric Cournand. At that time, Cournand was serving the position of a professor at the Columbia University College and worked at Bellevue Hospital in New York City. Cournand immediately understood the importance of the technique. He and his colleagues began to work on developing the ways of applying Forssmann's technique to heart disease diagnosis and research.

Cournand decided to make several alterations in the old catheters, including changes in the design and fabrication of tubing materials. Subsequently, he observed that *in-situ* placement of catheters in some patients for more than forty-eight hours did not cause any significant complications. By selective placement of catheters in different chambers of the heart, Cournand could collect true mixed venous blood. Due to this, the use of the direct Fick principle for the very first time became a reasonable means for measuring cardiac output.

Fick principle is mainly used to calculate the exact amount of blood flow to any organ by calculating the dissolved indicator in the blood. When one considers the heart, the amount of blood flow every minute becomes the cardiac output. The cardiac output can be calculated by dividing the uptake of the indicator by the content difference of indicator measured in arterial blood and mixed venous blood samples when the aspects such as the amount of indicator taken up by the organ per unit of time are constant, the initial concentration of the indicator supplying the organ, and the concentration of the indicator leaving the organ are known. Oxygen consumption was the indicator measured in Fick's original description for measuring cardiac output. Being able to measure cardiac output and the oxygen saturation of each of the cardiac chambers by selective catheterization was of great help as it delineated many complex structural heart diseases in a detailed manner. Moreover, the rate at which any medicine or intervention is helping an injured heart could be studied thoroughly by its effect on the rise or fall of the cardiac output.

André Cournand took the potential of catheterization created by Forssman to its logical conclusion by applying for the diagnostic and analysis of hemodynamics of the heart. Forssman, though a risk-taker and early innovator, lacked the resources for moving his research forward which was thwarted by the watchful eyes of conservatism. He did not have the financial backing, support of a larger institution, and manpower that Cournand was lucky enough to have. In collaboration with Dickinson Richards, Cournand performed more systematic measurements of the hemodynamics of the heart, which yielded tremendous success as well as peer recognition.

After a difficult span of prolonged isolation and humiliation, Forssmann finally received his due respect in the year 1956. The Nobel Prize in Physiology or Medicine was awarded to Cournand, Richards, and Forssmann. But unfortunately, Forssmann's entire career was spent in doing ordinary medical practice in unknown rural hospitals. After winning the prestigious Nobel Prize, he was offered a senior faculty position at a renowned research hospital. But Forssmann refused the offer politely knowing fully well about the progress of medical knowledge since 1929 when he made that "epoch-making discovery" in cardiac catheterization.

***

By the end of the 1950s, essential efforts had been mounted on the rising problem of coronary artery disease. Full concentration was given on medical research as post-war Europe and America had been facing disastrous deaths and devastations caused by the CAD epidemic. For any further work, it was crucial that the coronary arteries were adequately visualized as well as blockages quantified by a suitable diagnostic experiment. This method of diagnosis of CAD came to be referred to as "coronary angiogram". It was discovered serendipitously by Dr. Mason Sones, who was a pediatric cardiologist and researcher at Cleveland Clinic.

On October 30, 1958, Sones was working in the catheterization laboratory in his hospital. The patient was a twenty-six-year-old having rheumatic heart disease. As the first step of catheterization, he performed a left ventriculogram by placing a catheter into the left ventricular chamber. In the next step, Sones planned to pull the catheter out into the aorta and take an aortogram. This technique was used to delineate coronary arteries by nonselective contrast injections. The dye was imaged by X-ray waves released from an emitter device above the patient's chest, as it was radiopaque, and the entire procedure was captured by a recorder system. The results, however, were often not very helpful as a faint outline of the arteries were made visible. It was also observed that the surgeons had frequent difficulties in understanding the course and pathology or anatomy of coronaries at the time of looking at the films.

On that very fateful day, Sones waited a while, as he pulled the catheter back into the aorta, till the injector was being reloaded with 40 ml of contrast agent. His intention was to capture the picture of the aortogram next. All of a sudden, the catheter inadvertently slipped into the right coronary artery. Sones turned the camera on and was completely unaware of the situation. Before Sones could become aware and pull the catheter out of the right coronary artery, the complete load of contrast medium of 40 ml was directly injected into the large dominant right coronary artery. **When he became aware, chaos broke out as this was a 'terrifying moment" for both Sones and the staff present at the catheterization laboratory.** During those days, doctors believed that injection of dye directly into the coronary artery can bring about sudden death for the patient by causing ventricular fibrillation.

Fear engulfed the surroundings as Sones observed that the patient's heart had stopped beating. There was "asystole- the stoppage of heartbeat" for six long seconds and the patient was about to become unconscious. Applying great presence of mind, Sones asked the patient to cough. Fortunately, the pulse returned, and the patient regained vitals to everyone's relief. Sones then looked at the recorder screen. To his surprise and rejoice, he found that the injection was selectively visualizing the right coronary artery and its branches in beautiful detail.

"Being an experienced and thoughtful person as he always was, Sones brilliantly converted this terrifying and awkward mistake into an opportunity". From this nerve-racking incident, Sones realized that smaller amounts of contrast dye injected directly into coronary arteries are safe for the patient. But he had to be completely sure about it. Hence, he initially gave 10 ml of dye in a slower injection speed into the coronary arteries selectively. After various permutations on dose and speed, the final coronary angiograms became fruitful extracting excellent pictures of coronary arteries without any chance of complication for the patient. Sones subsequently did the selective cannulation coronary angiogram of almost a hundred patients, thus establishing it as a safe and useful procedure. Sones published his findings of more than fifty cases at the American Heart Association's Scientific Sessions in 1959.

Sones' perfection of "selective coronary cineangiography" brought about a transformation in the lives of millions of patients all across the world. Henceforth doctors could assess coronary obstruction severity by seeing accurate pictures of the blockages. Then they could advise appropriate treatment strategies to the patients. Any abnormalities of the vessels—such as plaques, calcifications, dissections, or clot formation—could now be studied in the minutest detail. It had elaborately defined the morphology of coronary patho-anatomy, allowed an accurate diagnosis as well as classification of coronary arterial lesions. Scientists could finally understand the natural history of coronary atherosclerosis. Subsequently, this innovation provided the stimulus for coronary artery surgery, also opening the path for percutaneous transluminal coronary angioplasty (PTCA).

Besides angiography, Sone's contributions in various allied fields are worthy of mention as these markedly improved the image quality and utilization. He and his expert team and skillful engineers developed X-ray generators, which produce short, square-wave pulses that can be synchronized with motion picture camera shutters; recording systems and closed-circuit television; use of cesium iodide phosphors to enhance image amplification; and, last but not the least, improved mechanical systems, facilitating patient comfort and allowing new projections. The "new generation of digital catheterization laboratories" available for cardiac interventions in modernized hospitals in the present era which work with immense accuracy and image clarity evolved after being benefited from Sone's excellent work.

Throughout his career, Sones was honored with several awards, including the American Medical Association's 1978 Scientific

Achievement Award and the Gairdner Foundation International Award in 1969. He was awarded the Texas Heart Institute's Ray C. Fish Award in the year 1973. For all his scientific discoveries and awards, Sones always held the strong belief that "he was a doctor first and a scientist later". His relationship with his patients was exemplary all throughout his time at Cleveland Clinic Cardiovascular Medicine Department. He headed the department at this hospital from 1966 to 1975. A quotation was kept in a frame in his chamber in Cleveland Clinic and it truly spelled what he meant, "I expect to pass through this world but once; any good thing therefore that I can do, or any kindness that I can show to any fellow creature, let me do it now; let me not defer or neglect it, for I shall not pass this way again."—Etienne de Grellet (1773–1855).

***

Gruentzig completed his training on public cardiovascular health in London and returned to Germany in 1969. He started working as a clinical fellow on May 1, 1969 at the Angiologische Klinik Germany, a hospital specializing in vascular medicine. While working there, he had to ponder upon a peculiar question asked by one of his patients. This question was so unique that his interest was raised and transformed his approach toward the treatment of CAD. The patient asked him that "instead of using drug treatment or undergoing complex coronary bypass operations, whether it was possible to just "clean" his obstructed arteries. In a similar manner, a plumber cleans tubes using wire brushes!"

Most scientists would laugh at this naïve question, coming from the simple mind of a patient; but Gruentzig found this idea, *"fascinating"*. From this very moment, he began to establish his first theories about therapeutic vascular interventions. He completely immersed himself in his ideas for building up safe and effective therapeutic options for arterial diseases. After some time once Gruentzig had been called to appear for a personal interview for the post of clinical fellow under Dr. Hegglin, the famous Swiss doctor. When Hegglin asked about his future plans Gruentzig said: "I have dedicated my life to vascular disease".

While working at Angiologische Klinik in Germany, Gruentzig once attended an afternoon lecture by the Frankfurt Vascular Medicine Circle. The whole program was organized by some of the leading vascular physicians of Germany of that era. During that afternoon, Eberhard Zeitler, of the Aggertalklinik in Engelskirchen, was requested to present his experience and clinical success by using the new Dotter angioplasty procedure for treating peripheral arteries of legs and arms with progressive catheter dilatation.

While concentrating on the lecture, Gruentzig felt that the procedure had significant potential for application on similar patients in his clinic. On his way back from the meeting, Gruentzig asked his department head H. M. Hasse, M.D. about the Dotter procedure. Hasse, however, curtly replied, "I will never allow this kind of technique to be practiced at my hospital". This was "a sign" to Gruentzig who had made up his mind to work in the field of vascular medicine. He soon decided to move to a newer job. He applied for a post of clinical fellow at Medical Policlinic at the Kantonspital of the University of Zürich. As soon as he was selected, he moved to Zürich. Gruentzig later moved to the Department of Radiology of the University of Zürich and started working under Josef Wellauer where he started conducting diagnostic angiographies at the hospital.

Meanwhile, Gruentzig continued to maintain contact with Zeitler and visited him at the Aggertalklinik frequently, thereby familiarizing himself with the Dotter technique. As mentioned, "Gruentzig observed the procedure keenly and saw the patients before and after treatment and when they left the hospital. He was very impressed with the improvement in peripheral ankle pressure as measured by ultrasound. He was impressed by the fact that the patient who came with severe pain in his leg due to obstruction of leg arteries was able to walk without any claudication after successful catheter treatment."

Gruentzig thought that it was high time he introduced the method at the University in Zürich. There was an angiology meeting in Lucerne,

Switzerland, in which Zeitler was supposed to give a lecture. As this was near Zürich, Gruentzig immediately grabbed the opportunity and requested Zeitler to come to Zürich with his catheters. Gruentzig promised him that he would provide him a suitable patient. When Zeitler agreed, Gruentzig invited his colleague radiologists from the Department to attend the surgery hoping that the whole team would feel motivated about the new procedure. "Unfortunately, this episode would end in a fiasco for Gruentzig'.

Gruentzig had prepared a patient with severe peripheral artery disease with claudication pain. The patient had severe stenosis in the proximal superficial femoral artery. Moreover, he had been studied angiographically for diagnostic purposes. A special laboratory was arranged for the surgery. Gruentzig assisted Zeitler while ten of his radiological colleagues observed them with keen eyes. Everything was as according to expectation until at the end of the procedure when the patient began to feel serious pain in his lower leg.

Gruentzig then realized that the entire plaque from the stenosis site had "embolized downstream" into the popliteal artery. The plaque had lodged at the bifurcation of the lower leg arteries and had obstructed the flow causing severe pain and discomfort for the patient. The radiologists who were skeptical from the very beginning, now had their proof that the method was of no use whatsoever in human beings. Gruentzig's attempt to convert his colleagues to the Dotter's technique ended in a failure.

Gruentzig's difficulties went on piling up as he had no state funding or scholarship to support him when he began indulging in his research work on the subject of vascular medicine. He had to complete all the routine jobs of the hospital as was expected of him besides finding extra time for carrying out his personal research. Putting aside all challenges, Gruentzig carried on with his work on the advancement of a new dilatation catheter and succeeded in performing his first peripheral angioplasty exactly four months later.

On February 12, 1974, Gruentzig, for the first time, applied his new single-lumen dilating catheter successfully with a 4-mm balloon in his patient. Fritz Ott, a sixty-seven-year-old, had been admitted because of incapacitating claudication of his leg, which was basically caused by severe femoral artery stenosis. After Gruentzig's angioplasty was successful, Fritz Ott was soon free of pain and was able to walk properly. This was followed by another angiography and Gruentzig performed a successful balloon angioplasty of femoral artery balloon dilatation just a week later. The patient was a seventy-four-year-old. These procedures thus provided Gruentzig confidence that he too had a suitable approach for the vascular stenosis problems. He did a series of peripheral angioplasties before venturing into the most complicated and risky part of the arterial stenosis, that of the coronary arteries.

Coronary artery dilatation had always been "the holy grail" of vascular nonsurgical intervention called balloon angioplasty. This later became renowned as PTCA, a brief acronym for a rather heavy-lifting label of percutaneous transluminal coronary angioplasty. Many clinicians, including Dotter himself, unsuccessfully held the dream of achieving the same result in coronary arteries just as they could achieve in the case of peripheral arteries. The most troublesome hurdle with coronary dilatation, however, was the catheters and other hard wares available during those days. The obstructions in the heart circulation needed a dilatation with uniform and reliable expansion so that it is not ruptured easily. For this, one required a small-bore catheter with a distensible segment; but the available balloon material could only be expanded around the lesion and did not provide the exact force necessary to open it.

Gruentzig decided to work with many versions of the balloon catheter which were basically designed and built with tiny bits of rubber, thread, epoxy glue, and so on. Unfortunately, none worked as per the expectations. At that moment, Gruentzig came to the conclusion that he needed different material than what was available to build his new catheters. The second vexing problem was the expansion of the balloon catheters. The problem remained the same no matter what—when distended in a constriction, the balloon always transformed into an "hourglass appearance", almost like a dog-bone, without opening the lesion.

The following two years Gruentzig immersed himself in research to find out a way to get over the balloon and material issues that plague coronary artery dilatation procedure. He thoroughly went through all the books on polymers and plastics, glues, chemicals, organic chemistry, and many more. He contacted numerous manufacturing units in an attempt to come up with a solution to this problem. Finally, he found a factory that produced shoelaces. They provided him with silk meshes that he would wrap around the balloons; this in turn it limits its outer diameter.

During his quest for the new materials to make the balloons work properly, he met a retired chemist. His name was Dr. Hopff and he was a professor emeritus of chemistry. Gruentzig was introduced to a new material, polyvinyl chloride (PVC) compounds by Hopff. From this Gruentzig was able to acquire some small thin PVC material that is used as insulation for electrical wires. In the next step, he began to experiment with this material. According to the instructions given in the descriptions in the books, he understood how to use the material. In the very beginning, he heated a localized segment of the tubing. Then he applied compressed air pressure which resulted in a localized aneurysm of the tubing. In the next step, he used a second outer tubing that measured 4 mm in diameter and began to confine the diameter of the inner segment.

Gruentzig had not been able to find a suitable place in the hospital where he could carry out the research work on coronary catheters in a proper manner. **Finally, having no other options left, he decided to use his small apartment as a makeshift lab. His kitchen table became the "test bench".** Oblivious to the apparent improbability of the place as a front-end research place, Gruentzig would often be busy on the small table late into the night with his materials, tubes, plastics and polymers spread all around. Gruentzig preferred using his kitchen stove when he needed to heat the polymers. His wife Michaela would later use this same stove for preparing dinner. When the catheters were completely ready and Gruentzig was satisfied with the outcome, he would take these to the hospital. Subsequently, he used these on his patient's legs after sterilization and later in their hearts. It can be safely stated that no cardiac research as big as coronary angioplasty which is hundreds of billions of dollars' medical industry today has ever been solved on a kitchen table as in Gruentzig's case.

For the next two and half years, Gruentzig prepared each balloon catheter "custom-made" for every individual patient. Prior to the PTA procedure, Gruentzig would obtain a native angiogram, take it home carefully and measure the arterial lumen and then the length as well as the width of the stenosis from the angiogram. From the measurements, he would calculate the optimal diameter and length of the balloon needed. Then he would build a balloon catheter to fit that particular stenosis. Gruentzig would accomplish this together with his assistant Maria Schlumpf and the help of their spouses, Michaela Gruentzig and Walter Schlumpf, Gruentzig being the only doctor in the "unknown ragtag team".

After hundreds of experiments and toiling for two tough years, finally Gruentzig was able to solve the shape issue. He observed and came to the conclusion that the sausage-shaped balloons worked at their best for uniform and consistent expansible force on the bench experiments. Then with the silk mesh, Gruentzig tried to reinforce the balloon surface. He suddenly realized that the strength of this material was so great that the silk mesh was not necessary at all. This happened when he mounted the material on a normal catheter tubing while applying pressure to distend the aneurysmal segment. This was a great breakthrough and enabled him to further reduce the size of the catheter.

The new balloon catheter made by Gruentzig is basically "a double-lumen dilatation catheter". It contains a main lumen and an additional lumen. The main lumen allows insertion of the guidewire, injection of contrast dye, and pressure measurements. While the balloon segment at the catheter tip can be positioned in the stenosed or occluded vascular segment and is filled with liquid by the additional lumen. The atherosclerotic plaque occluding the artery is pressed against the vessel wall for ten–thirty seconds by applying a constant and equally distributed pressure between four and six atmospheres. It is observed that the maximum diameter of the inflated balloon is 8 mm for iliac arteries and 4 mm for femoral arteries.

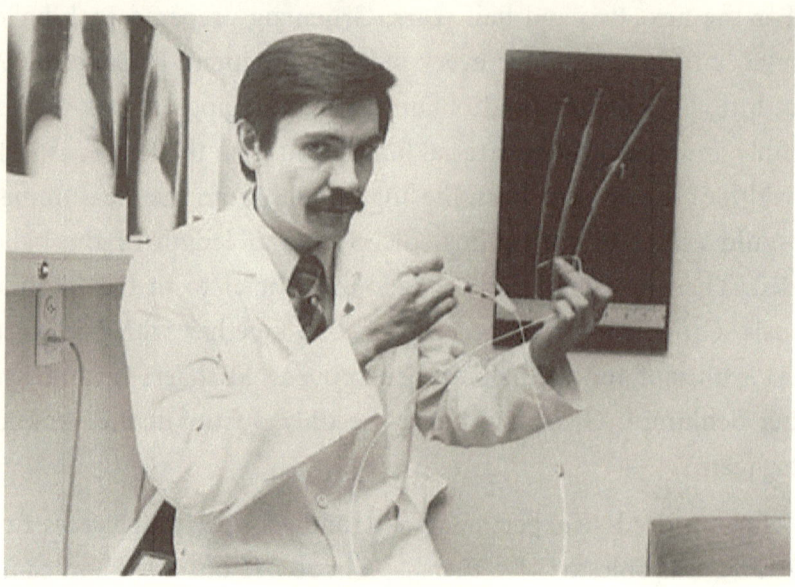

FIG: Andreas Grüntzig with his "double lumen balloon catheter" used in the balloon angioplasty for expanding lumens of narrowed arteries as a treatment of coronary artery disease

The newly formed vascular lumen opens as soon as the balloon is deflated, and blood flow is restored. The balloon will adhere to the catheter in its deflated form, just like an umbrella, and can be pulled back easily. Gruentzig's catheter stood out from the previous catheters made by Dotter and Fogarty because of its ability to simultaneously dilate at precise pressure as well as visualize and make hemodynamic measurements of the vessels while conducting the procedure. "This was a huge differentiator as the coronary arteries' intervention required precision and safety, which only Gruentzig's catheter was able to provide".

The second lumen over the Gruentzig's catheter required a completely separate plane for the dilatation procedure. But the access channel was not always satisfactory, thus making the balloon catheter too bulky to maneuver. After some tinkering, Gruentzig was finally successful in solving the second lumen problem in an ingenious manner. He constructed a miniature plane and was able to make a longitudinal groove on the angiographic catheter's outer surface. This was considered as a great step forward. Then he took a long PVC tubing with the distensible balloon segment on the end and slipped it over this angiographic catheter fixing at the proximal and distal ends.

Gruentzig also started to explore other vascular territories while continuing to treat patients with peripheral vascular disease by using advanced double-lumen balloon catheters. The catheters were still of bigger profile. In 1974, Gruentzig began to experiment and develop new techniques with catheters of reduced diameter that would smoothly allow their use in coronary arteries. But in the very beginning, he needed to experiment with the catheters in dogs kept in the experimental labs. He also required crucial support from a different specialty, that of cardiac surgeons, for trying his balloons in a real-life scenario. This was easier said than done as cardiac surgeons at Zürich Hospital were very "skeptical" about the whole experimentation.

The surgeons at the Zürich Hospital were unable to foresee the scenario of a complicated bypass surgery being replaced by an ordinary balloon catheter. They also were deeply worried regarding their patient's safety as they were scared of thinking about the catheter getting ruptured or entrapped inside the delicate coronary arteries of patients' hearts. Many important cardiac surgeons of Zürich such as Siegenthaler, Krayenbühl, and Hans-Ulrich Buff simply showed no interest in the procedure Gruentzig wanted to have on their patients. Finally, one surgeon came to the rescue of Gruentzig's plan. He was a cardiac surgeon called Åke Senning. Senning fully supported and actively helped Gruentzig to proceed further with his plans. In fact, when Gruentzig approached him seeking help and asked whether he could count on his support, he responded in his quirky humor, "Mr. Gruentzig, you will be taking away my patients, but get started right away!"

Gruentzig soon began to test the smaller balloon catheters for coronary arteries in lab animals as well as human cadavers. He ended up spending countless hours on this seemingly unattainable experimental research. One of the doctors assisting Gruentzig during that time was the Croatian cardiac surgeon Marco Turina. Turina had been commissioned by Senning for performing cardiac surgery in the experimental studies. In one of the interviews, Turina—while remembering Gruentzig's work ethic vividly—said, "He had the 'sacred fire', as the French call it. It was what he thought about constantly. I have never seen somebody so centered on a single idea like Gruentzig was. Never in my life. Everyone was telling him his idea would never work, and had been tried before, and that he was going to fail, that there were pitfalls at every turn. But the idea was consuming him all the time."

Gruentzig's younger daughter Sonja also recalled afterward about how she used to have her meals at the same kitchen table where the catheters were carefully made. **She smilingly joked about herself being a 'twin' of her genius father's beloved balloon catheter!** She would watch on with fascinated eyes as her father was completely immersed in making his idea work.

Gruentzig began evaluating advanced, thinner, and more refined coronary balloon catheters within the canine coronary arteries, within which earlier the surgeons had experimentally induced coronary stenosis. The first balloon dilatation of a coronary artery of a dog was performed in Zürich on September 24, 1975. Gruentzig collected all the data from these experiments. Then he decided to present it at a poster session demonstrating the efficacy and feasibility of this approach. He presented it at the American Heart Association's Scientific Sessions in Miami from November 15 to 18 in the year 1976.

Dr. Spencer King was present at the conference at Miami when Gruentzig presented his paper; he was one of the prominent cardiologists at Emory. At the exhibit section of the conference venue, King met Dr. Paul Lichtlen, Chief of Cardiology at Hanover. Lichtlen said, "You must see the exhibit by this man from Zürich in the next aisle." When a curious Spencer King arrived, he found Andreas Gruentzig standing in the center of a small group busy explaining his new balloon catheter. With his bushy mustaches quivering with excitement, he clearly was convinced that the method would work. **After watching Gruentzig's paper and explanation carefully for a great length of time, Dr. Spencer King observed wryly, "This will never work."**

Besides King, most of the cardiologists were also of the consensus opinion and believed "the device would never work". It was nothing but overconfidence and audaciousness to think that a flimsy PVC-balloon-coated catheter could dilate the hard and calcified gruel inside the diffusely diseased atherosclerotic plaque of the coronary arteries in a beating heart. More accurately it was also believed that the expanded portion of coronary artery plaque would immediately squeeze and recoil to its previous state the moment the balloon was removed, making the procedure futile and baseless. Gruentzig was the only exception who thought differently. He was the only lonely soul stuck in the research of one of the most important topics of heart disease. The improbability of Gruentzig's technique succeeding was gigantic. That is the reason why there was hardly any competing doctor, or even hospital, working on the technology in contrast to other promising topics such as valve surgeries where many universities and their medical teams worked simultaneously. For most researchers of his time, Gruentzig's work was like "an offbeat research of an eccentric mind".

As a famous quotation says, "Everyone knows that something cannot be done until someone comes along who doesn't know that it's impossible, and he does it." Gruentzig would soon proceed further to prove everybody else wrong. By the time he came back from the United States, he was determined to test its feasibility in a human study in coronary artery disease patients. To his misfortune, the first attempt of human angioplasty in the coronary artery misfired badly.

On March 22, 1977, Gruentzig finally had a chance to explore the feasibility of his new coronary balloon catheter for percutaneous transluminal coronary angioplasty (PTCA). The surgeons working in Gruentzig's hospital had a specific patient suffering from CAD. He was very symptomatic having severe chest pain. The angiogram displayed severe multi-vessel CAD, including a left main stenosis. The surgeons had already predicted the outcome and had declared the patient "inoperable". Hence, Gruentzig was invited to see if his new invention could help the patient.

Unfortunately, the operation began on an ill note. Gruentzig failed to gain femoral access—an approach required to reach the coronary artery ostium with the help of the catheter. Next, he tried by using brachial access. After a lot of effort, the left main artery of the heart could not be accessed. The procedure was hence abandoned. The patient died several days after the procedure of a final myocardial infarction. The first failure was a huge lesson for Gruentzig. **He later said, "The case taught me that if you start a method, you should start with an ideal case and not with end-stage disease."** This was his guiding principle in other similar cases that he faced later. This made him remember the dictum, "A surgeon is as good as the case he chooses to operate."

Gruentzig was not someone who would be haunted by a failure. He decided to refine his technique and safely apply it to the human coronary artery by performing the dilatation simultaneously with the intraoperative bypass surgery. He reasoned that any complication occurring out of dilatation of the coronary artery due to the balloon can be taken care of by the cardiac surgeons who are present at the operation theater. He tried to convince the surgical colleagues in Zürich for trying the dilatation in the patients. But these cardiac surgeons resisted the application of intraoperative dilatation as they feared that it would result in closure of the bypass graft. There were also certain elements of "turf war" involved in it. This was because the CAD patients till then had been entirely treated by cardiac surgeons. They would not find it palatable that a competing technique by fellow cardiologists be pushed into the forefront. As it often happens in the real world, surgeons of different specialties jealously guard their territory often refusing to collaborate with other fellow departments even while being faced with the logic for the benefits of the patient.

Discouraged by the "cold response" he received from the Zürich surgeons, Gruentzig began to search elsewhere. Fortunately, his cardiologist friend Dr. Richard Myler practicing at St. Mary's Hospital in San Francisco came to his rescue. Gruentzig had befriended Myler during his USA visit for a poster presentation. With Myler's help, Gruentzig was finally able to convince Elias Hanna, who was a cardiac surgeon at St. Mary's hospital, to assist them with this endeavor. Dr. Hanna agreed to the trial saying that his bypass grafts would "always be better than what was accomplished with dilatation."

Just like Dr. Hanna, most cardiac surgeons belonging to the first decade of angioplasty looked at the procedure with a benign disinterest. They thought it would always remain a poor cousin and a small adjunct to the bypass surgery. An assertion that would be severely tested in the following few decades as the competition between PTCA and CABG accelerated afterward. PTCA (percutaneous transluminal coronary angioplasty), which began as "an underdog" in the field of myocardial revascularization, saw a complete transformation in subsequent decades. It kept on refining itself with better balloons, wires, catheters, and other hardware in a continuous manner. This was spurred by innovations and helped by industry collaborations. In recent times, a vastly a greater number of patients suffering from coronary artery disease are treated by PTCA rather than bypass surgery, as patients are diagnosed earlier due to proper availability of diagnostic facilities.

On May 9, in the year 1977, Gruentzig along with Myler's assistance could perform the first coronary balloon angioplasty in an anesthetized patient during a coronary bypass surgery by retrograde insertion into a stenosed coronary artery right after arteriotomy. In each procedure, Hanna began the surgery by opening the thorax. Before establishing the aortocoronary bypass grafts, Gruentzig and Myler conducted several coronary balloon angioplasties on the diseased coronary arteries. Both of them continued with this procedure on several other patients. Gruentzig finally observed that all patients had a successful dilatation of the coronary obstruction. Moreover, he also found that none of the lesions developed any problem during the procedure.

Gruentzig was now confirmed and confident that he was indeed ready for "the real thing"—the angioplasty procedure in a native vessel in the catheterization laboratory without opening the chest. He returned from the USA as a confident individual and soon enough an opportunity arrived at Gruentzig's door for him to try his procedure.

***

Adolf Bachmann, a thirty-eight-year-old amiable Swiss insurance salesman, was admitted with severe precordial pain in the University Hospital at Zürich. His angiogram revealed a solitary discrete lesion on the proximal part of the left anterior descending artery (LAD), which is the largest branch of the coronary vascular system. The lesion was much severe and could easily block the blood flow leading to angina. The doctors advised Bachman for bypass surgery. Bachmann was hesitant to undergo the rather extensive surgery. Then he got to know about "the new technique" of nonoperative procedure called angioplasty. It was at this moment that Bachman got to meet Gruentzig regarding the issue. In the meeting with Bachman, Gruentzig revealed all the difficulties while discussing the procedure. He even disclosed in front of Bachman that his procedure had never been done before in the world, so there was a risk of having an emergency bypass operation.

Bachman, however, was determined to undergo the new procedure. Bachman once told in an interview that "the way Gruentzig truthfully and elaborately discussed the procedure with him made him decide for going ahead with the technique". What followed afterward is history.

On September 16, 1977, on a Friday early in the afternoon at a time when the anesthesiologist and the cardiac surgeon were available and no cardiac procedure was underway in the operating room, Gruentzig brought Bachman into the catheterization laboratory. Bachman was catheterized by taking a femoral access from his groin by putting a small needle assisted keyhole opening on the femoral artery. Gruentzig proceeded with the surgery, while the Chief of Cardiology, the cardiac surgeon, anesthesiologist, cardiology and radiology fellows keenly observed him from the recording room.

Gruentzig positioned the guiding catheter retrogradely up into the aorta and then was placed in the left coronary orifice. In the next step, the dilatation balloon catheter was inserted through the guiding catheter. A roller pump was on standby to assist in coronary circulation in case the blood flow ceased during or after balloon dilatation. This was basically done to make the arterial blood available for pumping in via a roller pump through the main lumen of the dilatation catheter into the coronary artery to "perfuse the myocardium" during the balloon inflation. It was observed by Gruentzig that this technique was effective for preventing acute ischemia at the time of coronary experiments done on the dogs.

On the fluoroscopy, Gruentzig was able to see as the balloon reached the occlusion site. The balloon was inflated as soon as the catheter wedged to the stenosis. When the balloon went up to full pressure, Gruentzig vividly noted that "there was no sign of any antegrade flow and simultaneously the distal coronary pressure was very low". **At that moment, Gruentzig and the team watched breathlessly to see if there**

was any development of complications. Most of the clinicians expected the complication related to the sudden cessation of blood flow to the LAD artery leading to hypotension, shock and ventricular fibrillations. Many others dreaded the possibility of a coronary artery rupture as the plaque edges were fragile and calcified than normal coronary wall.

However, no ST elevation, ventricular fibrillation, or even extra systole occurred which surprised everyone. The "most amazing thing" during the procedure was that Bachman remained conscious throughout. He even did not feel any chest pain! Watching the clinical status of Bachman, Gruentzig finally decided not to take any help of roller pump for the coronary perfusion. Moreover, right after the first balloon deflation, the distal coronary pressure rose nicely. Encouraged by this positive response, a second balloon inflation was conducted to relieve the residual gradient. After the second dilatation, Gruentzig carefully removed the balloon catheter and took an angiogram shot to observe the LAD coronary artery. The flow to LAD was satisfyingly spontaneous without any obstruction while Bachman peacefully stayed on the table completely conscious. Everyone was surprised about the ease with which the procedure was rounded up. Suddenly, it dawned upon Gruentzig that "his dream of so many years" had come true.

Gruentzig published the results of coronary balloon angioplasty as a preliminary report in *The Lancet* in the year 1978. He published the results of a much larger number of cases together with Senning just in the following year. By April 1979 Gruentzig had treated sixty patients by applying PTCA. Most procedures went smoothly without any hitch like Bachmann's. However, a few did face hiccups. Six patients had to undergo emergency bypass surgery to prevent a major myocardial infarction. A few of these patients had to experience a myocardial infarction. However, all these patients survived the PTCA or the surgical procedure.

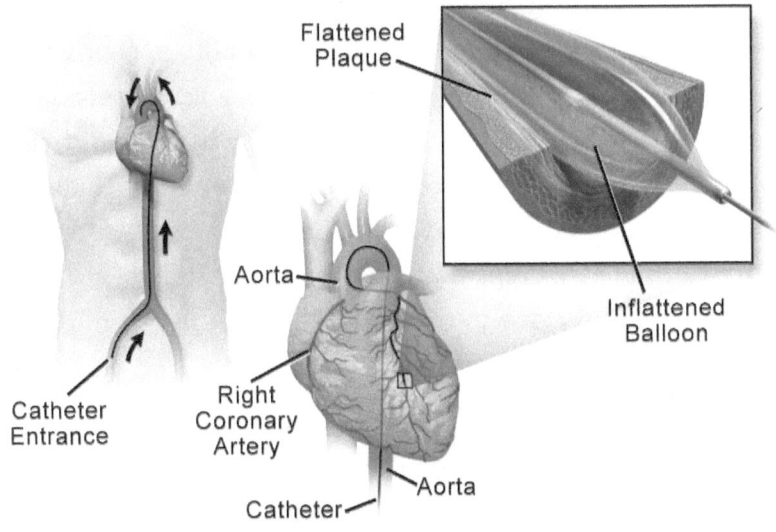

Balloon-tipped Catheter

FIG: Balloon angioplasty procedure with balloon catheter inside the coronary artery

By April in the year 1979, Gruentzig reported a primary success of PTCA in forty-one out of sixty patients. To be precise, this success is quite less when compared to the recent standard which is well above 90% success. "At that time, however, it created seismic waves amongst the cardiologist scientific community". It was a miracle to witness a person survive a heart attack and be relieved of severe angina pain without even having the chest opened for bypass surgery. Furthermore, there was no need for anesthesia and the patients undergoing angioplasty were comfortable being awake or being under minor conscious sedation. There was huge interest in Gruentzig's method among the medical fraternity. **Patients from all across Europe and America approached Gruentzig asking him to conduct the miracle operation on them.** Soon other doctors began to follow the trend. PTCA was soon successfully applied on patients by Richard K Myler in San Francisco, Simon H Stertzer in New York City, and Martin Kaltenbach in Frankfurt.

In the 50th Scientific Sessions of the American Heart Association's (AHA) meeting, Gruentzig got another opportunity to choose between presenting an update of the dog experiments in a verbal session similar to the previous year and reporting on the first patients treated by angioplasty. He decided to choose the latter course and asked for an early one-month restudy of the first patient. During the AHA presentation, he arrived completely prepared with a summary slide of the first four patients treated. In the history of Heart Congress, this became one of the most memorable presentations ever.

Gruentzig's presentation of the PTCA angioplasty at the conference was attended by learned cardiologists from all around the globe and they gave stunned acknowledgment to the doctor's hard work. Gruentzig showed all the four cases done successfully elaborating Bachmann's case right at the very beginning. The results were there in the form of grainy black-and-white angiography images. It was one of the greatest historical moments being observed by everybody. At last, Gruentzig displayed the slide of the fourth patient with the incredible success of the main stem of left coronary artery dilatation, which was "the riskiest procedure" to conduct even with a bypass surgery and an open chest. It was during this case that the audience started applauding impressively in the midst of the lecture. Gruentzig was so surprised that he was almost unable to proceed with the ten-minute presentation. He was engulfed with shapeless emotions. His years of hard work had finally paid off. Moreover, his dream of seeing CAD patients being treated in the simplistic novel manner was appreciated by experienced cardiologists from far and wide. The same doctors who had earlier ridiculed his audacious thoughts and rash attempts now were keen to learn the technical aspects from Gruentzig. They were not disappointed. Gruentzig would teach everybody his new method in a "most open and transparent manner ever".

On February 4, 1978, Gruentzig's report of the first five PTCA patients' cases appeared in the prestigious medical journal, The Lancet.

Four days later the Zürich Newspaper Tages-Anzeiger published a front-page article, displaying a photo of Gruentzig and Siegenthaler with the headline "Zürich's important contribution to fighting myocardial infarction." The article was followed by a press conference that was broadcasted by the Swiss national television. Less than a week after the press conference, the local German newspapers also had praised the new procedure immensely. On February 13, 1978, Lichtlen, the same doctor who had said Spenser King to watch Gruentzig's poster at AHA conference in Miami, wrote a personal letter to Siegenthaler, with a copy to Senning and Gruentzig:

"...I consider your approach of informing the public at the present state of this technique with only ten treated cases und unknown long-term results as very premature and therefore of most questionable value. Hopes which currently by no means can be fulfilled were created among many patients..."

Fortunately, time would tell that Lichtlen's concerns were not justified. The number of angioplasty (PTCA) cases not only increased over time, but also it became a most useful technique by fulfilling the aspiration of patients to be treated in a noninvasive way relieving symptoms and saving innumerable lives. By the mid-1980s, more than three hundred thousand PTCAs were being performed on an annual basis, and these equaled the number of bypass surgeries being conducted for CAD. By the year 1990, lumen stenosis of the coronary arteries was more frequently treated by the angioplasty technique than by surgery. One reason for such rapid adoption of such a revolutionary and totally advanced approach was because of Gruentzig's working manner. His passion for teaching and sharing knowledge was utmost strong just as his desire to innovate the growth of this nascent technique in many countries in a fairly rapid manner.

Following the success of the PTCA, vascular medicine and cardiology colleagues from all across the continents arrived in Zürich hoping that Gruentzig would teach them the new method. Such a huge number of trainees could not be allowed into the operation theater all at once. Finally, Gruentzig decided to start a "live demonstration" course at the Zürich Kantonsspital while performing balloon angioplasty in the catheterization laboratory. From then on, Gruentzig held various live demonstration courses in Zürich between 1978 and 1980, which were mainly attended by vascular physicians and cardiologists from America, Europe, and Asia.

Gruentzig sincerely and selflessly wished that this technique could be used for humanity's benefit as widely and universally as possible. His live demonstrations were the most interesting and unique thing in the training of any medical surgery, later tried and adopted by other specialties. While the procedure was being carried out in the catheterization laboratory, hundreds of eager cardiologists would be staring at the screen sitting in a next room auditorium with bated breath completely mesmerized by the new technique. Gruentzig would move to and fro between lab and auditorium while explaining, discussing, and analyzing. Afterward, he would say that a number of these discussions actually clarified his own doubts. He could conduct the next operations in a better manner. **It was the humility of a great mind, who never felt small to share or learn.** Countless times he had to face many fiercest of critics as a proponent of any advanced technology would. But his calm demeanor, charisma, and persuasion would win over everyone. At the end of the intense debate, he would get a wide round of applause and come out triumphant.

Although the angioplasty (PTCA) method had just been introduced into clinical practice, Gruentzig did not consider this a problem to perform it live in front of the watchful eyes of fellow visiting doctors. According to his former assistant Maria Schlumpf, Gruentzig was very much convinced about its safety when it could be performed with perfection. She said, "Once somebody asked Gruentzig why he chose to perform in that way at the early stage, as a live case with direct CCTV transmission of the surgery."

Gruentzig had an honest answer, 'If the method is good, it should work even in a live demonstration. If not, let's look at it before we endanger our patients!'" It was this type of teaching which directly confronted a critical as well as an enthusiastic audience with the truth and which helped a great deal in teaching and spelling out the method.

Gruentzig repeatedly emphasized on avoiding complications and ensuring patient safety both in his procedures and his teachings. According to him, this has the utmost priority while selecting patients for coronary balloon angioplasty. **His deepest concern regarding patient selection or a procedure was his belief that every patient is also a grandmother, a husband, or a son to somebody. His love and respect for his patients and concern for their well beings were abundant.**

Many years later, Gruentzig gave his very last interview with Burt Cohen in which he expressed his concerns about the safe use of his invention in the future. He said, "It is easy to be a hero and do a lot of dilatations and a lot of stenoses, but you also then have to be a hero to face the family in which you feel that probably the approach wasn't right and should have waited a day instead of getting in and trying to elegantly do everything in one session and running into trouble which could have been avoided. So, if you want to be a hero, you better be it also in the follow-up and when you face the patient's family after you had a trouble."

The journey Gruentzig started from the University of Heidelberg in Germany to lead to the successful invention of angioplasty at Zürich was about to take another turn. Despite the overwhelming success of his new treatment, his home institution and his superiors were skeptical and unwilling to provide him with the required support. While patients were queuing up to avail angioplasty at the only place in the world where it was available, they had to wait a long time. Siegenthaler, the Physician-in-Chief of the Medical Policlinic, would allow Gruentzig only two operations per week. On the other hand, there were hundreds of helpless patients waiting desperately with several serious symptoms of chest pain and cardiac failure.

Faced with the moral dilemma, Gruentzig tried his best to approach several other authorities to seek help for his patients. But he was stuck in between the hierarchical system of the University Hospital, and it was not at all easy to get a solution. Thus, Gruentzig had no other option but to watch helplessly as the PTCA list kept on growing. Many patients on the waiting list were having their stenosis close completely, getting heart attacks, and dying. This was a terribly sad moment for Gruentzig. He could not remain silent while his patients deteriorated in front of him, more so as he knew he had "a solution" for these unfortunate patients. He started to look for opportunities outside his hospital.

Being completely aware of his talent, various other institutions, among them Harvard University and the Cleveland Clinic, offered Gruentzig secure positions. Through his acquaintance with Spencer King, John Douglas, and others at Emory, Gruentzig finally met Dr. William Hurst, the Chairman at Emory University in Atlanta, GA, USA. Gruentzig liked the offer from Emory and accepted Dr. Hurst's invitation to join his team. He then became a professor at Emory University Medical School, with the understanding of serving as the Director of Interventional Cardiovascular Medicine.

At Emory, Gruentzig's adventure began again. His initial years at the new workplace was like a dream run. He was much relieved and felt liberated from the rigid environment of Zürich and thus looked forward toward blossoming to his full potential. While previously he used to perform two angioplasties a week, he did the same numbers in a day at Emory. Over a span of five years, he was able to perform more than two thousand eight hundred coronary angioplasties without losing a single patient. Being a keen observer, he was able to improve in a rapid manner with each passing month and the results displayed his success.

Within no time, the learners flocked to the Emory campus to get a firsthand experience of angioplasty from the master trainer. He sponsored an annual postgraduate course attended by hundreds, published numerous quality research papers, and propelled cardiology at Emory to the top ranks of world medicine. **Between 1980 and 1985, Gruentzig was able to organize ten of his famous courses for his colleagues who arrived at Emory traveling from all corners of the world just for receiving his advice.** His professionalism as a clinician as well as his excellence as a teacher was a rare combination indeed. J Willis Hurst, one of the most prominent faces in the history of cardiology, describes him as "Gruentzig was a genius. While he loved life and lived on 'the edge', he was a tender, honest, and compassionate advocate for his patients."

However, Gruentzig's work and life happened to be brief at Emory. The year 1985 was disastrous for major pioneers of interventional cardiology. Melvin Judkins died from myocardial infarction in January. This was followed by the death of Charles Dotter who succumbed after a second coronary artery bypass surgery in February. Finally, Mason Sones died of lung cancer in August. Hence, Gruentzig alone remained: 'the only survivor' among the early pioneers. Tragically, Andreas Gruentzig's life ended all too soon. His second wife, Margaret Ann, and he met their death in his private airplane that crashed on October 27, 1985, while flying between Sea Island and Atlanta, Georgia.

Gruentzig's best quality was his perseverance against all odds. He had enormous will power, intellect, optimism and diligence, but never changed or succumbed to pride. Hurst described him as "a real Mensch" in 1986. He said, "What a role model he was! The greatest stimulus to learning is the behavior of another person who exhibits noble attributes. Everyone who knew him realized he was unique. As each individual discovered his great attributes, he or she became a better person. This, I believe, was his greatest teaching achievement."

Unfortunately, Gruentzig did not live long enough to see the "true impact" of his breakthrough procedure. PTCA or coronary angioplasty was destined to completely transform the way cardiology was practiced. It was unthinkable that from being the persons who only diagnosed coronary artery disease and let the cardiac surgeons take care of the blockages, the cardiologists would be able to treat the root of the problem themselves. A paradigm shift occurred gradually with an increasing number of patients availing of the noninvasive technique of PTCA over bypass surgery (CABG). The biggest strength of angioplasty was the simplicity of the procedure. The standardization of procedures with required consumables such as catheters and guides could make it available to almost every corner of the globe. Gruentzig's unselfish and open manner of live teaching method was followed up by his trainees. This in turn helped in spreading the novel technique to Asia, Middle East, Africa, and Latin America.

The industry medical collaboration was a crucial cause for the expansion of angioplasty and the advancement of hardware. Even a serious situation like a critical left main obstruction at the origin of the coronary artery could now be treated in a catheterization laboratory, rather than an open-chest bypass surgery. It was really surprising to see a patient walking out of the catheterization laboratory in a short span of ninety minutes after getting angioplasty done; to top it all he could be discharged and join work the very next day. But there were many unsolved technical issues, and one knew that solving these would make Gruentzig's technique the procedure of choice for most cases of coronary obstructions. One common problem was "dissection or abrupt closure" of coronary arteries during or after balloon angioplasty. Such an unwelcome event often caused a heart-attack-like situation on the operating table. This in turn required urgent bypass surgery.

Just a year after Gruentzig's death in 1986, Puel implanted the first self-expanding coronary stent on March 26, 1986 at the University Hospital in Toulouse, France. The second operation was conducted by Ulrich Sigwart in Lausanne on June 12, 1986. The stents were metal scaffolds; these were basically a "tiny wire mesh tube", created by LASER cutting. It props open an artery; then it is left there permanently. Initially, they were designated as 'coronary endoprosthesis'. Then in 1987, Julio Palmaz and Richard Schatz implanted their balloon-expandable metallic stent into a patient in Germany. Stents took care of the dissection and abrupt closure complications of PTCA and made the procedure much safer and predictable. From that moment onward, Gruentzig's angioplasty advanced and improved to achieve its "true potential".

***

Gruentzig's legacy, pioneering spirit, and passion will live on in the hearts of many cardiologists and innovators through the continued evolution of what the great genius created. He became the inspiration for many biomedical scientists and doctors across the globe. In recent times, angioplasty has the capacity of saving thousands of lives every year. Building on the use of balloon catheters for restoring blood flow in stenosis, coronary and peripheral arteries angioplasty have developed into one of the most successful therapeutic interventions of all time.

Angioplasty developed at a rapid pace throughout the early 1980s with multiple innovations. In 1982 steerable guide wires were developed at the request of Gruentzig and others. This, in turn, dramatically improved the ability of reaching distal segments of the coronary tree. Meanwhile, with the introduction of very-low-profile balloon materials that allowed "high-pressure inflations", catheter development continued; the horizons of angioplasty were further expanded. By 1984, angioplasty could display enough growth and advancement for testing it against bypass surgery. Several trials were conducted to decide whether bypass surgery is a better option than PTCA or vice versa. But the debate has not yielded any definite conclusion till date. **At present, both bypass surgery and angioplasty remain the most viable options for treatment of Coronary Artery Disease, in turn complementing each other frequently.**

Gruentzig understood very early that a lot of new things were to be discovered and superior techniques invented to achieve the final destination of the procedure which he had successfully introduced. Gruentzig once said in an interview that he was working on some new gadgets and techniques for improving angioplasty. His mind was already fixed on the "next big thing" in coronary intervention. Many other contemporary cardiologists of Gruentzig's era believed that he would have pioneered several other techniques had he not met with his untimely death. Joe Brown, Dr. Gruentzig's chief technician, remembers him as a man always interested in finding answers. "'There are no problems,' Gruentzig would say, 'without solutions.'"

Although most new devices had their evolution in the late 1980s, several of these advancements were ongoing before Gruentzig's unfortunate death. One such was the "LASER technique" of coronary angioplasty. In fact, Gruentzig experimented with laser therapy in Zürich before arriving in America. It is even recorded that he also worked with several other devices to open coronary arteries. Another of the most interesting methods was the procedure conducted with the drilling machine. This consisted of a thin elastic wire, and its distal end was bent into an elliptical form. Its proximal end was connected to a "rotating drill" with the distal end in the artery at a speed of 3000 revolutions per minute. The wire developed the form of an ellipse, similar to that of an eggbeater, while spinning and displaced the atherosclerotic material against the arterial wall. Then in April and July of 1972, the device was tested in animal models. However, Gruentzig's pressing work with balloon catheters interrupted further advancement of this procedure.

Later, Gruentzig techniques found a place in modified form among several innovative plaque removal techniques called atherectomy devices as an adjunct to balloon angioplasty coronary interventions. These include the utilization of the excimer laser for photoablation of plaque, directional atherectomy for cutting and removal of plaque, and rotational atherectomy (use of a high-speed diamond-encrusted drill) for mechanical ablation of plaque. Such devices are useful in decreasing the incidence of restenosis in selective cases when used as an adjunct to standard percutaneous coronary intervention. Excellent improvement of coronary artery imaging such as intravascular ultrasound (IVUS), optical coherence tomography (OCT), and fractional flow reserve (FFR) has also contributed to better therapeutic results of PTCA.

Since the first angioplasty was conducted, newer and better techniques as well as gadgets have been invented every year adding a new way to reduce coronary stenosis. Many of the techniques have remained for a few years and disappeared gradually as they could not stand up to rigorous clinical trials for showing additional benefits. On the contrary, some have remained in use. The original balloon angioplasty, however, remains the mainstay of treating coronary artery disease. **The idea to use the natural vascular system of the body as the therapeutic highway for balloons, catheters, medicines, and stents to cure or modify CAD is considered the most original thought ever in the field of cardiology.**

After Gruentzig's renowned success of coronary angioplasty aided by Dotter and Fogarty's foreknowledge, the new branch of medicine—interventional cardiology—achieved its true potential. From that time onward, it has grown to become one of the commonest procedures performed in hospital stays. Over the past twenty years, the use of angioplasty has increased rapidly in most countries. Around the mid-1990s, it gradually overtook coronary bypass surgery as the preferred method of revascularization—about the same time that the first published trials of the efficacy of coronary stenting came to the forefront. In recent times, angioplasty now accounts for 78% of all revascularization procedures and is equal to or exceeds 88% in Korea, Estonia, France, and Spain and other OECD countries. It is recorded that each year over 965,000 angioplasties are conducted in the United States.

***

It was 4:30 in the morning when my mobile screamed relentlessly, waking me up. From years of working experience as a medical professional, I know that the awkwardly timed calls are never to deliver happy news. As I picked up the phone, I found it was Dr. Prabhakar Babu, the Director and CEO of our hospital, on the other side.

"I have a friend from Hyderabad who has just landed at the airport. He called me to say he has some chest discomfort. I have told him to reach the Emergency Department. Can you please take care of him?" Dr Prabhakar spoke.

As I parked my car marked as 'only for emergency doctors' at the front of the hospital—a 12-story tall glass façade in the heart of Visakhapatnam, popularly called city of destiny—the early morning chill of December was still in the air. Soon I walked into the emergency room. Dr. Manoj, the doctor on duty, told me it was a case of acute anterior wall MI. I picked up the ECG from the file. In a sharp upstroke, the ink markings on the ECG had gone up several notches and extended to all his six chest leads on ECG, which is a sign of serious ischemia leading to a heart attack. The person, whose name was Srinivas, had come to Visakhapatnam city on a business trip. He already had a five-star hotel room booked for him. When he called Dr. Prabhakar from the airport, he told him that he would prefer to go to the hotel, take a shower, and would come to the hospital for a checkup. Prabhakar had wisely directed him to first come to the emergency for getting a quick ECG on the way. "This tiny bit of advice became a life-changing experience for Srinivas".

As I walked toward the bedside to meet Srinivas, a 50-year-old suave gentleman, he was very apologetic about giving trouble to me in an early morning errand. "It must be the food in the flight," he said. "I am already feeling slightly better, after taking the tablets given by your duty doctor. I think half a day's rest at the hotel will be ok for me."

"Self-denial" is the biggest cause of cardiac complications. Even in places having the most sophisticated hospitals in the developed countries—like in Europe and the US—many thousands of people die each year because they refuse to call 911 Emergency Help number as they fail to realize that any chest discomfort may be serious. I spent a few minutes to tell him that I had already seen the ECG which was indeed of a very serious nature. We had to proceed with an emergency angioplasty procedure to handle the massive clot which had built up inside his coronary artery and was killing thousands of his heart muscle cells every minute.

As an educated and reasonable person, Srinivas caught the gravity of the situation in my counseling. His friend and our CEO Prabhakar's call came soon after convincing him on the matter. I told the ER staff to shift him immediately to the Cath Lab as I proceeded upstairs to get the operation theater rolling.

Only five minutes had passed, and I got a call, as I was changing into the operation theater dress. This time from the anesthetist, Dr. Rao. "The patient had a fibrillation of heart while being shifted to transport in the lift. His heart arrested and there was asystole for about ninety seconds. We have shocked him, intubated, and put on inotrope." It was simply the worst news I could have ever received. Fibrillation is when the heart descends into a chaotic aimless quivering effectively leading to complete cessation of pumping. A few minutes of ventricular fibrillation can cause permanent and irreversible brain damage. Out-of-hospital cardiac arrests have a dismal survival rate of 3%–4%. Even though Srinivas had developed ventricular fibrillation inside the hospital with immediate attention of medical personnel thanks to his agreeing to come down to the hospital directly from the airport, it was still difficult to predict how much of his myocardium had been completely knocked off. I felt sorry for the gentleman.

I was already scrubbed and waiting when Srinivas was wheeled into the Cath Lab. He was unconscious under atracurium and midazolam; a tube was hanging from his mouth connected to a portable ventilator delivering oxygen to his lungs. As I watched him, it was difficult to guess if any neurological damage had occurred to him after the arrest or not.

Without wasting any more time, I proceeded with an angiogram which showed the proximal LAD coronary artery was completely occluded with a clot. The big artery which supplies 70% of circulation to the heart in normal times was completely cut off right at the origin!

Srinivas was suffering from "widow-maker heart attack". It is an informal term used for those heart attacks which carry the highest risk of death. Usually, the left main or proximal LAD coronary artery is completely obstructed with a thrombus in 'widow-maker heart attack' causing a huge loss of circulation to a large part of the heart. This in turn leads to electrical arrhythmia, asystole and death by cardiac arrest.

I soon passed a guiding catheter through the groin into the aorta exchanging for the diagnostic catheter. Through the guide catheter, an ultrathin metallic-coated wire was passed from the aorta into the coronary artery crossing the obstructed path. Thereafter, another smaller catheter with multiple holes at the tip was passed over the wire into the clot-laded artery. Under the fluoroscopic X-ray guidance, the clot is sucked out from the coronary artery through the catheter. The material, when put on a white gauze piece, looked like tiny cheese pieces dipped in tomato sauce.

The coronary blockage was further cleaned by another balloon dilatation with additional clot-busting drugs given directly into the problem areas. Finally, a stent—a coil of a metallic alloy of 30 mm length—was implanted to restore Srinivas' blood flow completely. The procedure lasted for about forty-five minutes. All the time Srinivas remained "immobile and unconscious" while being watched over by the anesthetist across the table.

After three months, I saw Srinivas again as he walked into my OPD. He had lost some weight and his face showed signs of fatigue, probably due to the exhaustion he had to undergo during his last stay. But in every other way, he was absolutely normal. Any person, who is unaware of his medical history, would not be able to guess looking at him about his recent tough battle.

Srinivas hailed from Hyderabad, a city with world-class cardiac care facilities, from where he traveled to Visakhapatnam for the sole purpose of his medical follow-up with me. He was the director of a business house. He needed to travel to Hong Kong on an upcoming business trip for which he wanted my permission. More than his stated objective I believed he visited us to reinforce his feelings and make his confidence grow by visiting the place which saved his life.

As I saw Srinivas' echocardiogram and other reports, I told him he was absolutely fit to do any physical exertion or traveling as he wanted. Both of us probably shared the same amount of satisfaction and relief with the outcome of his clinical problem. As he was about to get up collecting his prescription, Srinivas asked one thing which was probably inside his mind for long, **"Did my heart stop that day, doctor?" A question so forthright, most people will not even dare to ask their doctors.** "Yes," I said looking into his eyes, which were moist with a new hope.

***

After the operation's success, Srinivas was able to get discharged from the hospital after a few days. He could walk out on his own, unaware how greatly he had been benefited by Gruentzig and the other cardiologists' innovations in this treatment. Before coronary angioplasty, the only way for a heart attack patient to remove the clot and restore flow in his coronary artery was to give blood-thinning medications by injections and then helplessly wait, hoping for the best. In this method, called "thrombolysis", the success rate for restoring blood flow was only 50–60% compared to more than 90% by angioplasty procedure when carried out within 90 minutes of the patient being presented in the ER.

During the last meeting with me, Srinivas curiously asked about the reason "he was having this problem while being a nonsmoker, vegetarian as well as with no prior medical history of heart disease". We could not provide him with any specific reason. **"Srinivas is similar to many of those people who fly below the conventional radars designed to red-flag risk patterns"**. The doctors still find it difficult to explain why some people who have apparently no reasons to fall prey to heart attack risk calculated by traditional risk factors do have one.

In spite of all the development in this specific field, the exact time and cause of myocardial infarction and the potential sufferer has not been possible to predict till date. "Thus, this lets CAD maintain its mysterious aura". New developments—one in the field of coronary calcium analysis and other on the study of genetics—however, may give an answer to this most intriguing question: 'Who among the thousands of apparently healthy people are going to get a heart attack and who is going to be spared of the dreadful event?'

One useful way to assess the probability of developing coronary artery disease in the future is to do a "coronary calcium measurement" by CT scanning. This severity can be presented numerically as coronary artery calcium (CAC) score or Agatston score.

The Agatston score got the name from its developer Arthur Agatston, a clinical professor of medicine at Florida International University. This score is basically a measure of calcium on a coronary CT calcium scan. The original work was based on electron beam CT also known as ultrafast CT or EBCT. The score is calculated using a weighted value assigned to the highest density of calcification in a given coronary artery. The density is measured in Hounsfield units, and a score of 1 for 130–199 HU, 2 for 200–299 HU, 3 for 300–399 HU, and 4 for 400 HU or greater. In the next step, this weighted score is multiplied according to the area in square millimeters of the coronary calcification. Let us take an example. A tiny spot of coronary calcification in the LAD measures up to 4 square millimeters. It basically has a peak density of 270 HU. Therefore, the score comes to 8 (i.e., 4 square millimeters × weighted score of 2). It is also observed that the tomographic slices of the heart are 3 millimeters thick. It has an average of about 50–60 slices from the coronary artery ostia to the inferior wall of the heart.

The summation for the calcium score of every calcification in each coronary artery for all of the tomographic slices is done to know the total CAC score. It is seen that on the basis of the fact that calcium present in coronary arteries can lead to the accumulation of plaque, this risk calculation methodology is used to decide. Over the years, this calcified substance can cause atherosclerosis or a narrowing of the arteries. It is vividly observed through experimentation that atherosclerosis restricts oxygen supply and blood flow to the heart. This will potentially result in a massive heart attack or drastic stroke.

It is seen that the CAC score is an independent marker of risk for cardiac events, all-cause mortality, and cardiac mortality. Moreover, it provides additional prognostic information to several cardiovascular risk markers. Even in the present times, many heart attacks continue to occur in people who are considered as low or intermediate risk. This is because the traditional risk models are not much useful in predicting heart attacks. It is also seen that in determining an individual's risk, coronary calcium scoring is proving to be a game-changer in all sense.

While the coronary calcium score is a rather wide and population-based method for predicting heart attack, the most immediate query in everyone's mind is, 'is it possible to do it better by more accurate and individualized analysis?' Moreover, is it even possible to predict heart attack risks before any drastic damage has already happened? This is specifically crucial and as it is cited by CT coronary calcium scan with the calcium deposit method, the damage has happened by the time when the heart has already developed early changes of plaques. Surprisingly, one may claim that all these answers can be found in our genes, which are the universal codes within every human being. **Our genes preordain a lot of things about ourselves including 'when' and 'how' an artery might rupture to form a clot within the delicate surface of the heart.**

The genetic factor is proving to be an important element of causality of coronary artery disease as heart disease is mostly found in family clusters. If somebody's father or grandmother had a heart problem at a particularly early age, then it is highly likely that he might develop the same disease as well. Said that, we are not entirely hostage to our genes. "Heart disease is more of a combination of nature and nurture effect. That means a lot depends not only on what genes do to us but also what we do to our body. Regular exercise, a healthy diet, and being a nonsmoker is also important to reduce the chances of heart disease".

Over a decade or more, researchers have been using genome-wide searches to unveil genetic clues linked to heart disease risk. It is like a very large puzzle where each genome is like one piece of it. These markers, called SNPs — "single nucleotide polymorphisms', are single-letter changes across the genome that vary from person to person There are millions of spots on the genome, which, when taken individually, convey only a minor information about cardiac risk. But taken together, they can be grouped to better predict the disease. In genetics parlance, these groups are known as polygenic risk scores (PRSs). Some researchers have used these risk scores in a similar way that single-gene variants can predict cancer or the unusual high-cholesterol disorder called familial hypercholesterolemia.

The idea of using an individual's entire DNA sequence for predicting heart disease got a massive boost from an advanced study that successfully used the method. The study used the genetic assessment PRS, which looks at many variations in DNA that influence disease. Using PRSs is considered one of the most promising advances in heart disease research. A study presented in the AHA's journal *Circulation: Genomic and Precision Medicine* looked at a group of people—in this case, French Canadians. Lead author Guillaume Lettre, who was a professor at the Montréal Heart Institute and Université de Montréal in Canada, has pioneered a study undertaking the detailed genetic analysis to find PRS patterns in the people studied. To powerfully predict the future cardiac risk, the study observed 3639 French Canadian adults with CVD and 7382 adults without heart disease. The study vividly displayed that the scores can identify 6%–7% of people at high risk of cardiac disease.

Early detection could help the doctors to quickly choose simple, effective treatment such as aspirin, statins, or other medications. The next step logically would be for large clinical studies for determining whether treatment based on risk scores can improve the patients' heart health or not. In addition, researchers sometimes need to determine how to integrate the scores with known risk factors, such as blood pressure, diabetes, and cholesterol levels. Researchers also require extending these studies to non-European ancestry populations. Everyone hopes the day will come in the future, when a simple and cheap genetic testing from a swab of one's saliva will give us all the information which is hidden under the complex genetic helices.

If rapid progress is made in making the genetic studies sharper, we may be able to personalize medicine by hunting down bad gene carriers and treating them aggressively. Maybe it will take some more research and rigorous work to finally "turn the clock back". The insights into basic molecular mechanisms gained during the era of interventional cardiology will definitely bring us closer to the ultimate goal of eliminating coronary artery disease as a major health risk one day. **The pinpoint accuracy of the genetic fault line and their clinical correlation remain a "work-in-progress" till today.** Hence, Gruentzig's angioplasty combined with medicines and lifestyle change remains the best answer to coronary artery disease for the time being.

***

Summer of 2019 is the time for EURO PCR conference at the massive convention center at the Palais des Congrès de Paris—VIPARIS, in Paris. It is one of the most important events on the calendars of interventional cardiologists worldwide. One of the world's largest congregations of interventional cardiologists from Europe, Asia, Africa, and America has arrived at the center to learn, collaborate, teach, and celebrate the developments in the field of cardiology. The technique of open and live demonstration and interactive way of learning traces its pattern to the ways which took its origin from Gruentzig's angioplasty workshops four decades back. This is one of the biggest events held annually where cardiologists gather to share their experiences and often candidly "admit mistakes" while carrying various interventional procedures including coronary angioplasty.

The discussions at the conference follow the long tradition established since the time of Gruentzig himself of being open, transparent and registry-based approach: to seek the truth amidst a growing number of gadgets, wires, balloons, and plaque-busting devices brought out annually by various research groups. The sprawling conference venue is a few hundred miles away from Gruentzig's center in Zürich where he brilliantly conducted the first coronary angioplasty of the world, launching the branch of coronary intervention.

As part of the program agenda at the international cardiology conference, "a live satellite transmission" of a cardiac angioplasty procedure is taking place from a hospital in TEL Aviv—a city in Israel—to the conference venue. All the doctors seated in the auditorium are able to see in real-time the details of the procedure on the two giant screens displaying the live transmission in the main arena. This is a very immersive experience as multiple cameras inside the operation theater in the faraway city bring the minutest details of cardiac surgery as it progresses live.

Under the keen eyes of thousands of enthusiastic doctors, the operators are carrying on with angioplasty by balloons and stents as well as newer gadgets which are designed by different innovators year after year to make the procedure better, safer, and more successful. This is a "never-ending quest" to attain perfection. Sometimes these procedures can be nerve-racking for the operators like a live sports arena with the challenge of time and tension of being successful in front of the global audience.

Despite the complex clinical case and operative challenge, the TEL Aviv operators complete the surgery with a perfect result. As the final angiographic shot is taken, the impossibly knotted coronary arteries are seen to be flowing with natural ease. And soon a broad smile appears on the primary operator's face with the audience joining the scene with a huge round of applause. While giving a thought-provoking explanatory demonstration, the operator-doctor gives his rich tributes to Dr. Andreas

Gruentzig for the discovery which saves thousands of heart disease patients' lives every minute in any part of the world today. This is exactly how Gruentzig would have loved it to be. With calmness in carrying out and explaining complex interventions while still having an adrenaline rush, "risk-taking came naturally to this charming doctor".

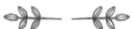

CHAPTER 4

ANGELS OF THE HEART

Hominem ad deos nulla re propius accedunt quam salutem hominibus dando. (In nothing do men more nearly approach the gods, than in giving health to men)

— **Marcus Tullius Cicero 106-43 BC**

A Prayer on the Lips

It was in the month of August, 1945 that Mrs. Edenburn arrived at Baltimore from Waterloo, Iowa with her gravely ill son, Hugh Michael Edenburn who was just at the tender age of two and a half years. The city of Baltimore is located about forty miles northeast of Washington D.C., the capital of the USA. Founded in 1729, the city carries with itself a significant part of the nation's history. Baltimore's Inner Harbor was once the second leading port of entry for immigrants to the United States. Afterward, the city became famous as a major manufacturing, heavy industry, and transportation hub as well as the rail industry. The busy Northeast Corridor of the passenger rail system passes through this city. Baltimore is the largest and most populous city in the state of Maryland.

Mrs. Edenburn looked "anxious and exhausted" when she arrived in this big city. Baby Michael looked even frailer. Grossly underweight, he helplessly had to be carried on his mother's lap. But the most striking fact about him was the color of his skin. Michael's lips were oddly purplish in color. His fingers and toes were deep purple in shade almost like blue. Doctors at the local hospital in Iowa had told Mrs. Edenburn that her son was suffering from a heart disease which was present in him since birth, a condition the doctors would label as "blue baby".

Being a white American child, Michael Edenburn's look would be striking to people at any other place with the contrasting color of his lips, nose and fingertips. But at these times in Baltimore, local people would hardly notice such an unusual phenomenon. The reason being the whole city had been recently flooded with blue babies who were accompanied by their parents.

It was amazing to see such a journey of hopefuls. Sick children from all corners of the United States and even from outside the continent would be streaming through the Penn Railway Station of Baltimore to finally reach their destination, the Johns Hopkins Hospital.

Recently, a piece of news had circulated that the doctors at the Johns Hopkins had found a new surgical treatment for the blue babies. Before this surgery became available, the diagnosis of a blue baby or cyanotic heart disease was the worst message about the child any parents could expect. One-third of all the babies would die within three years, and about two-thirds would not even live to see their tenth birthday.

A few other babies, who survived, would lead a life of torture and drudgery. They could hardly indulge in any worthwhile effort. Most never attended school or dropped out helplessly. On the playground, these children would feel "humiliated" as they would be breathless and unable to catch up with their friends who ran away from them. Over the years their growth would be stunted and their heights would be poor. With each effort becoming a punishment, it was as if they had a life sentenced for death.

The landmark surgical event occurred in the year 1944. World War II was raging transatlantic and all across Asia during that span. America had joined the Allied forces after the Pearl Harbor bombing by Japan. At that time, Franklin D. Roosevelt was the President of the USA. IBM had just launched a machine called Mark 1, a computer of the size of half a football field which would take up to three minutes to do a simple calculation of mathematics. The black enlistees were accepted by the US Army, but they created a completely separate black infantry regiments and then white commanders were assigned to them. The Negro units were given more menial jobs on the ships by the navy. Black and white soldiers were kept apart at the training bases and were "segregated by color".

News those days traveled leisurely. Airplanes were few in numbers and were used mostly for mails and war material transport. Civilian transport was mostly conducted by automobiles or rail. Crossing the Atlantic from America to Europe would take days on ships. Many important events and discoveries would take decades to be known or adopted at other institutes or countries. **Yet, this was such a remarkable lifesaving news that media all over America reported about this, in spite of being busy in war-related matters.** One day while relaxing at her Iowa home, Baby Michael's mother Mrs. Edenburn was reading Collier's Magazine. Suddenly her eyes got fixated on an article. She came to know about this miracle treatment at the Johns Hopkins Hospital in Baltimore, Maryland.

Baby Hugh Michael was born to middle-class parents at Waterloo, in the state of Iowa, in 1942. Within a few months of his birth, the doctors told Mrs. Edenburn that her child was "not expected to live to reach school age". **He was born a "blue baby"—a child with a malformation of the heart where the blood circulation to the lungs is restricted leading to insufficient oxygenation of blood.** This is a birth defect which affects hearts many unfortunate babies, of which Michael was also listed.

Day by day, this hole and a constriction in Michael Edenburn's heart were robbing him of energy, breathing, and life. When he started his baby steps, his mother noticed that after running around for a while he would sit down in a peculiar manner folding legs and arms. It looked like a "squatting position". He preferred to sit in that position because, after very little exertion, the blue coloration of the skin increased further which would make him dizzy. The doctors explained later that this peculiar position of squatting was because of him trying to save some oxygenated blood going to limbs so that it could be directed to the brain and other vital organs. A few times Edenburn would even collapse when the blood circulation to the brain decreased substantially. **These episodes of "fainting spells" were very alarming for his parents. During these spells, Mrs. Edenburn noticed that his fingers and toes would become deep blue from purple.**

With very little hope at the home state, Mrs. Edenburn decided that she had to go to Baltimore to save her son's life. From Collier's report, she knew about the surgery; it was devised by two hardworking doctors—Dr. Alfred Blalock and Dr. Helen Brooke Taussig. They were the two pioneers whose names are written in the highest levels of pediatric cardiac surgery history. What she and most people at that time would not be knowing about was a third person. This person, whose name was not mentioned in that surgery, had an equal if not more contribution to the discovery of this technique. This man was a poor black person from Nashville and was the grandson of a slave. He would overcome the "centuries of barriers of color" to give humanity the success to treat the poor babies with a surgery which was hitherto not humanly possible. His name was Vivien Thomas. Among them, the three pioneers would "change the medical history and defy many medical gospels."

After reaching Johns Hopkins Hospital, Mrs. Edenburn entered the main entrance that was beautifully adorned by a giant statue of Jesus Christ. She filled up the forms at the desk, completed all the formalities, and Michel Jr. was registered to be seen by Dr. Helen Taussig, the Chief of Pediatric Cardiology at this hospital. Soon Baby Michael and his mother were ushered into her chamber. Upon seeing Dr. Taussig, Mrs. Edenburn felt a strong sense of hope and positivity that had eluded her since Michael was born 2½ years back. Dr. Taussig's quiet demeanor and confidence was a morale booster for the emotional mother as well as everybody else at the pediatric wards. Taussig gently examined Baby Michael in her usual meticulous manner. Then she picked up her clinical notebook registry and noted down on a blank page: "Michael Edenburn, blue baby #44". From there onward, Michael would be logged into a journey hitherto taken by only a few similar of his conditions guided by the compassionate hands of Taussig.

***

Helen Taussig was born on the 24th of May, 1898, in Cambridge, Massachusetts, and was the youngest of four children. Her father, Frank Tausig, was teaching economics at Harvard University. Taussig's mother had been one of the first female graduates at the Radcliffe College, where she had studied biology and zoology. To the misfortune of the Taussig family, she died of tuberculosis when Helen was only eleven years old.

Mother's death was a big blow to Taussig's personal life. Her father, however, raised her with a lot of care, affection, and attention. While at school, she had a bout of flu for which she took medication. Afterward, she noticed a typical problem; "her hearing ability had decreased to a certain extent". Taussig became partially deaf which unfortunately continued to progress alarmingly.

Taussig doubled her efforts to keep up with fellow students. But unexpectedly, her school grades started to deteriorate gradually. Then one fateful day, her father noticed her not being able to form or join words to create sentences. She could neither read sentences properly nor comprehend them at all. It was then discovered that she had a serious problem of dyslexia, a learning disability. **Anybody else would give up hope against such adversity. But Taussig was a determined girl and her father was a very compassionate individual.** He decided to be by her side and help her in every possible way. He would be with her for hours and days so that Taussig could improve on her reading and writing skills. Finally, their wish was fulfilled and Taussig completed her school successfully.

After completing her school studies, Taussig followed in her mother's footsteps and chose to study at Radcliffe College in the year 1917. She got excellent grades in her studies. She developed an interest in sports and became a tennis champion in college sports. Two years later, she left for Berkeley University in California. There she successfully bagged her baccalaureate degree in 1921.

Afterward, Taussig wanted to continue her education at Harvard University, a dream she had nurtured since long. She had enough academic credentials for this. But Harvard in those days did not look at academic credentials of all impartially. In fact, Harvard did not even consider females worthy of entering its hallowed portal for the quest of education. It was not until 1945 that this male bastion officially allowed women to study medicine on their reputed campus. This was really disheartening for Taussig. The "motherless, partially deaf, dyslexic girl" would sit down to wonder what she would do next. **Often our destiny is controlled by the times we live in, but then one must have the courage to beat all odds.** Tausig was too brave and focused to be disheartened by situations like these.

Taussig decided to go to Boston University's Medical School where she could study biology and anatomy. Boston allowed girls to study, though practical classes for females were separated from the male students in those days. Taussig was assigned to write a thesis on the muscular bundles of a cow's heart. This work gave her motivation, and she became interested in the human heart afterward. She delivered an excellent thesis which was praised by her guide, Professor Alexander Begg.

With Professor Begg's encouragement, Taussig proceeded to take up medical studies at the Johns Hopkins Medical School in Baltimore. It was one of the few American universities that allowed women to study during those days. After obtaining her M.D. in 1927, Taussig took up pediatrics as a specialty. She also continued to develop a special interest in "pediatric cardiology, a study of children with heart defects".

Pediatric cardiology is a difficult subspecialty of cardiology. At that time, there was very little understanding about the mysterious conditions of congenital heart disease. There were neither any confirmatory tests available nor was there any textbook which could guide doctors to a particular diagnosis. The children Taussig saw were underweight and whining most times. The babies had a miserable life full of suffering and complications. There was simply no treatment for these conditions. Most doctors wisely avoided the subspecialty knowing the poor prognosis and resultant disappointment.

It is commonly known that a child's suffering is different from that of an adult's. The distressed baby in its pure heart does not follow etiquette. He will cry, groan with pain or yell at everybody to show his displeasure.

He will not try to be polite in pain like a grownup. On being relieved from misery, he will jump away with pure joy and play around. He will often forget to show gratitude. But a caring doctor like Helen would only feel the appreciation intuitively from his boundless joy and abundant smile. Taussig loved all babies—"ill or well".

As there was no diagnostic facility to detect cardiac malformation, the doctors in those tumultuous days needed three things: "knowledge of the normal and abnormal heart sounds, a stethoscope, and a good ear". Taussig was short of hearing due to her illness during her school days. As her deafness progressed, she would initially use a hearing aid and an auditory amplifier on her stethoscope. But soon she learned to use her fingers to feel the heart sounds. She could listen with her fingertips. It was an "amazing ability" and she became very proficient in this unusual skill.

Taussig excelled in her diagnosis with just her fingertips, which others had taken great effort to auscultate with ears and finest stethoscopes. Her colleagues would be mesmerized to find the absolute same diagnosis or even better when Taussig gave them the answer. She would go around pediatric wards feeling the babies' chests. Her slim fingers would be lying tenderly on the tiny children's chest while she would soak in information which her nonfunctional ears could not provide to her brain. "It was as if the girl from Massachusetts had learned to never give up".

Taussig was not only a good clinician but also a "curious scientist". She would meticulously label and organize all the pediatric cardiac problems which she encountered while seeing the patients. Equipped with her clinical skills and probing mind, an electrocardiograph, a chest X-ray machine, and a fluoroscope, Taussig began to collect samples and create a registry. In this way, she gained extensive clinical experience caring for children with congenital heart disease. She would correlate the pathology and clinical presentations with basic diagnostic tests available back then. She had a gift of putting up questions in a "stepwise manner" leading to self-evident answers. This is an attribute of a great scientist and teacher.

In the mundane years of the 1930s, such a specialty of pediatric cardiology was nonexistent. There was not enough understanding of heart ailments of children and their etiology. No serious textbook existed to guide the doctors into diagnose cases. Taussig would often make her own diagnosis by analysis and logical reasoning. Her notes in those years and later would come to be the foremost textbook of pediatric cardiology in the whole world. "In a way, she was her own teacher and the sick babies with cardiac disease were her sole textbooks".

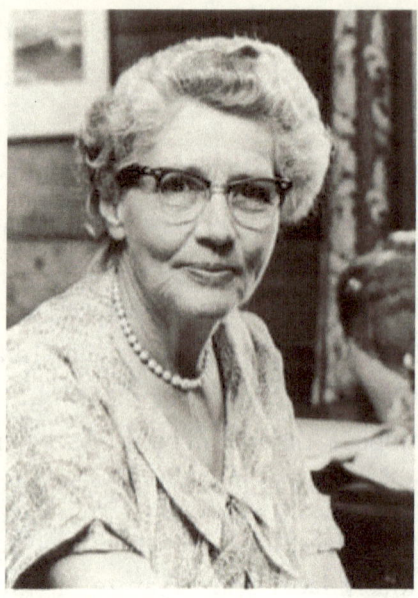

FIG: Helen Brooke Taussig. She is credited with developing the concept for a procedure that would extend the lives of children born with Tetralogy of Fallot, the most common cause of the blue-baby syndrome.

The Mystery of Blue Babies

In her pediatric practice, Taussig frequently saw babies with one peculiar problem which really captivated her attention. It was those babies who looked "blue" during and right after the delivery. After every act of milk sucking from their mother's breasts, they had to gasp for air. Even if they were given oxygen, the color or condition would not improve. It is called "cyanotic condition of a child", which presents because of reduced amount of oxygenated blood in their circulation. When the reduced hemoglobin is more in the blood, it manifests externally as cyanosis, a bluish-purple hue of the skin. In these babies, there was a congenital malformation, a defect in the structure and anatomy of the heart. Because of a narrow pulmonary artery, too little blood flows to the lungs, unlike in the normal condition, where it is abundantly provided with oxygen in usual cases.

In the normal human heart, there is a combination of "dual circulation" of blood running in series. They are called the systemic and the pulmonary circulation. The blood from the heart circulates in the body by going from the left ventricular chamber to the aorta and henceforth into systemic circulation. By the time the blood has come back to the heart again, it has given up most of the oxygen to the organs. This deoxygenated blood enters the other circulation through the right ventricle that is pulmonary circulation. At the lungs, the blood is again recharged with oxygen. Breathed in air present in the alveoli of the lungs carries oxygen which enters the blood cells at the same time the carbon dioxide is removed and exhaled from the body. This oxygenated blood now enters systemic circulation through pulmonary veins and via the left ventricle and aorta it is ejected out into the body. It is important that the left and right heart circulation remains separate as it is like "chemicals lying in experimental jars in the lab". If mixed up, the composition and utility of the oxygen-carrying hemoglobin in red blood cells will change which is unsuitable for the human body.

In "Tetralogy of Fallot" or the "classical blue-baby syndrome", this arrangement is disturbed due to structural defect of the heart present since birth. Even though many doctors had earlier described about this, Étienne-Louis Arthur Fallot, a French physician, was the first to describe the condition in detail; thus he is the one whose name the disease carries. Fallot used the name "La maladie bleue" (the blue disease) to describe the condition.

In 1888, Fallot described the "four anatomical characteristics" of Tetralogy of Fallot. Out of the four separate cardiac deformities, two are responsible for the characteristic skin pallor. The first of these is pulmonary stenosis, which causes narrowing of the exit from the right ventricle. The second is a ventricular septal defect, which is a hole in the wall separating the two ventricles. The third component of Tetralogy of Fallot is right ventricular hypertrophy or thickening of the right ventricular muscle. The very last of the four defects is a wrongly positioned aorta, arising because of deviation of outlet ventricular septum, which allows blood from both ventricles to enter the aorta.

In a Fallot "blue baby" child, there is a communication between two chambers of the heart due to the septal defect. Oxygenated blood from the lungs mixes freely with the blue, deoxygenated blood from the rest of the body. At the same time, the blood flow passing through the lungs is reduced substantially because of the narrowing of the pulmonary artery. When the heart contracts in Tetralogy of Fallot patients, a portion of deoxygenated blood from right ventricle passes to the narrowed pulmonary artery. But a major part of it crosses the ventricular defect and enters systemic circulation. What follows is a "combination of reduced blood flow to the lungs reducing oxygenation and mixing of deoxygenated blood with systemic blood".

Because so little of their blood could travel through the lungs, blue babies have extremely low blood oxygen levels, causing breathlessness, stunted growth and the unhealthy coloration which typifies the condition. During the period of exertion or anxiety like prolonged crying, pulmonary artery passage become narrower by spasm of the ventricle chamber outlet below it, deepening the blueness. Often during these periods of extreme reduction of right ventricular to pulmonary blood flow, the babies suddenly collapse, a condition known as 'Tet spells'. The color of skin already purple would turn deep blue at those spells. Many children die during prolonged spells.

Though Fallot's heart disease was known since the beginning of the twentieth century, the detailed anatomical analysis and pathophysiology were poorly understood. Dr. Taussig had kept this condition as the "A-list" among all of her problems and wanted to solve it with priority for it was the commonest causes of cyanotic heart disease or blue-baby in children at birth afflicting one in every 2000 babies born. Taussig made a detailed registry of all the cases with a record of severity symptoms and the time of onset since birth. She also kept fluoroscopic investigation and electrocardiogram of babies for comparative analysis.

One peculiar variation of presentation of Fallot's blue babies really surprised Taussig to a greater extent. But why was it that some of these babies died soon after birth, while others survived for months or even years? Even the color of the babies varied. Some were deep blue to purple. Some others were of almost normal color with a slight tinge of blueness on their lips. A few were of truly normal color and were termed "pink Fallot". The last group of babies would go unrecognized unless sought in detail.

Taussig guessed that there would be a pattern in the presentation. A special vessel caught her attention: "the *ductus arteriosus*". This is a short connection between the pulmonary artery and the aorta. In the normal babies before being born, a ductus arteriosus is a normal and essential shunt as the lungs are not ready to function. The shunt loses its functional utility as soon as the baby is out of the mother's womb. It closes down spontaneously in matters of days or weeks. In a few of the children, however, the ductus persists. This is a "harmful condition", stealing blood from systemic circulation through the shunt. This shunt is needed to be closed surgically to make them normal.

In contrast, however, in the blue babies, this shunt had the "opposite effect". Taussig noticed that those blue babies whose ductus arteriosus was patent after birth had a better result than those whose ductus closed spontaneously. The babies with a patent ductus were clinically better, with less cyanosis and a better survival record. Taussig, to be sure, kept on checking repeatedly the blue babies' clinical data as well as many cadaver postmortem reports which were easily available as the death rate was so depressingly high. Every time "a distinct pattern emerged"; blue babies born with a good-sized and functional ductus between two major arteries had better clinical and survival record. **Taussig started to believe that this ductus, while harmful when present in otherwise normal babies was important for Fallot blue babies to survive.** She thought if the shunt could somehow be kept open or a new artificial shunt was created in that place, it would definitely help the blue babies.

Tausig needed to prove "her theory" by application in an experimental lab or on operating table. Without proof nothing is valued at all. This was like entering a "never explored world" of heart surgery, which was quite a challenge. For this, she needed a surgeon who could create such a shunt. At that time, there was a famous surgeon in faraway Massachusetts, who was practicing in Boston Children's Hospital and was conducting a surgery involving ductus. But the objective of his surgery was the opposite of Taussig's study. He was able to close the ductus arteriosus of the babies who were born with patent ductus. His name was Dr. Robert Edwards Gross.

***

Gross was the son of a Baltimore piano-maker. He was born with a congenital cataract, and thus he could see through only one of his eyes. The defective eye remained unrepaired till the time when Gross retired from his surgical practice many decades later. As a boy, his father would give him smaller and smaller clocks to take apart and reassemble, training his depth perception and turning him into a finely skilled mechanic.

After graduating from the Harvard Medical School, he was trained in pathology, where his work in the laboratory and autopsy studies exposed him to many of the congenital heart malformations that were fatal at the time. He then completed a residency in general surgery at the Brigham attained the post of the Surgical Chief Resident for Dr. William Ladd, the Chief of Surgery when Lorraine Sweeney, a 7-year-old child, came to see him.

Lorraine grew up in Boston in the 1930s and was the youngest of eight children born to Irish immigrants. As a child, she was weak and tired easily, and her parents noticed a constant "buzzing" that seemed to come from her chest. Though doctors suspected that she had congenital heart disease, no effective treatments were available at that time. In response to her daughter's increasing debilitation, Lorraine's mother brought her to Boston Children's Hospital, where they met the young surgeon, Robert E. Gross. After examining Lorraine, Gross concluded that she had a patent ductus arteriosus (PDA) and that he could repair it.

Surgery on the heart, however, was not yet practical in 1938, though many earnestly hoped that operating on the great vessels could be the path for opening up this possibility. Surgical correction of a patent ductus arteriosus (PDA) was suggested as early as 1907 by Dr. John Munro of Boston, who demonstrated an approach via a sternal incision in infant cadavers. If feasible, ligation of a PDA could save many children from progressive heart failure and/or endocarditis. Life expectancy for this condition did not typically exceed late adolescence. Dr. Elliott Cutler, Surgeon-in-Chief at the Peter Bent Brigham Hospital in Boston was also examining the potential for surgery on the great vessels. He predicted that the first procedure might be the correction of a PDA. However, surgical ligation was not attempted until the year 1937, when an emergency procedure was performed by Dr. John Strieder at Massachusetts

Memorial Hospital on a 22-year-old woman with endocarditis. The patient survived the operation but died several days later.

When Gross asked Lorraine's mother, Mary-Ellen, for permission to proceed with the operation, she sought advice from their parish priest, who advised them by saying, 'Leave it in God's hands'. That is when Lorraine's family gave consent for the surgery.

There was a "serious obstruction" to Gross's plan to operate on Lorraine's heart. Dr. William Ladd, the Chief of Surgery of Boston Children's Hospital was not in favor of the surgery, since the only other previous attempt on PDA surgery had failed with the patient dying four days after the surgery. Ladd refused to grant Gross permission to perform an operation, telling him, "At my hospital, you will not perform such an operation!" As per the protocol of the department, Gross had to have permission from the chief to be able to proceed with the surgery. Gross, however, found a way out to outmaneuver the order. The legend has it that as soon as Ladd left for his annual summer vacation to Europe, Gross managed to get the desired authorization from his deputy, Thomas Lanman.

The operation took place on August 26, 1938. An incision was made on Lorraine's chest in the 3rd intercostal space on the left side, and the 3rd rib was retracted upward. The left lung collapsed, revealing a PDA that was 7–8 mm in diameter and 5–6 mm in length. Gross rested his finger on Lorraine's heart; then he simply described 'a thrill of extreme magnitude' that he felt over the pulmonary artery, but he even noticed that it kept disappearing over the aorta. **"When the [sterile] stethoscope was placed on the pulmonary artery, there was an almost deafening, continuous roar, sounding much like a large volume of steam escaping in a closed room."**

After the cardiac anatomy examination was completed thoroughly, Gross neatly wrapped a silk tie around the patent ductus arteriosus (PDA) and patiently waited. Lorraine's blood pressure shot up from 110/35 to 125/90. With this good sign on record, Gross performed a simple ligation of the duct. When the thread was tightened, the thrill over her heart disappeared, and the continual "buzz" from her chest was silent. Gross wrote in his operative note that the room all of a sudden seemed to become completely still. It had taken a little over an hour, and Lorraine was feeling quite energetic and healthy within a few days. Ultimately, the procedure was a great success, Lorraine going on with a healthy life till the age of 88 years raising her two sons and being a grandmother. Robert E. Gross made history in 1938 to become "the first surgeon in the world" to successfully ligate a PDA.

***

When Taussig mulled over her plan to meet Gross, he had already become famous all over the world by then and was consulted about any duct-related surgery. By that time, he had also done many successful PDA surgeries since the first case in 1938. Taussig traveled all the way from Baltimore to Massachusetts to meet him and discuss her hypothesis in detail. She requested him to elaborate if he could consider creating a shunt between the pulmonary and systemic circulation. That was basically to create a ductus arteriosus like structure artificially to help in cardiac circulation in the blue babies.

However, Gross was in a fix and was not at all sure if the technique of creating a shunt in the blue babies by connecting a systemic artery to a pulmonary artery would work or not. He light-mannerly said that he had enough trouble closing ducts; he casually rejected Taussig's proposal saying, "he did not want a new complicated issue of creating ducts". This remark of Gross would prove to be the most foolish thing he ever said in his entire life. Gross would dearly regret missing the chance of creating history later. Taussig returned with a heavy heart and was very disappointed.

After this rejection, Taussig decided to approach another surgeon who had been newly appointed at the Johns Hopkins at the very same time. He had joined there as the Chief of Surgery, Professor, and the Director of the Department of Surgery of the Medical School. He rightly attained fame at the young age of just forty-two years. He had got the top job at Hopkins due to his excellent research while previously working at Vanderbilt University. His name was Dr. Alfred Blalock.

Innovators and pathbreakers are rare in any age. Their true contribution can be measured adequately as a surgeon, scientist, or researcher when looking back in the mirror of history. Dr. Alfred Blalock was one such in the history of the long journey of medical science. Many have considered him the Father of Modern Cardiac Surgery. He was the one performing the first blue-baby operation in the world which is considered a landmark. Most medical historians agree that this single act of novel cardiac surgery made a giant leap into modern pediatric cardiac surgery possible.

Alfred Blalock was born on April 5, 1899 in the small town of Culloden, Georgia. This place is located in Monroe County in Central Georgia. It was a small community in a remote isolation of approximately 350 people. Blalock was the eldest of five children born to George Z. Blalock and Martha Blalock. George Blalock was a businessman and owner of a cotton plantation. He always cared for his children's education. Blalock always admired his father for the foundation he got in his early childhood.

At the age of fourteen, Blalock entered as a senior at Georgia Military College, a preparatory school for the University of Georgia. Shortly after, Blalock attended the University of Georgia for higher studies. He was outgoing and socially interactive at college. Being an avid sportsman, he was athletic and excelled in tennis and golf. He also was a secretary and treasurer of his senior class. After graduating with good grades in 1918, Blalock joined The Johns Hopkins School of Medicine.

During attaining his medical degree, Blalock enrolled for the surgical course on a rotation. "He was immediately in love with scalpels and sutures". He realized that this was where his career lay. He excelled in surgery and tried to get a surgical residency after obtaining his medical degree in the year 1922. But a surgical residency at the Johns Hopkins was very competitive; and Blalock, despite his best effort, could not obtain one. He had to accept a urology internship instead. In the following year, he earned an Assistant Residency on the General Surgical Service. This was then followed by an externship in otolaryngology in 1924.

Blalock moved to Boston in the summer of 1925 and decided to continue surgical training at the Peter Bent Brigham Hospital. Within days, however, he received a telegram from Vanderbilt University. The telegram mentioned that "Dr. Barney Brooks, the Head of Surgery at Nashville, had offered a position of Chief Surgical Resident to Blalock". Blalock immediately left Boston to move to Vanderbilt deciding to accept the offer. This incident and his decision became the turning point of his career.

Blalock completed his Chief Residency years at Vanderbilt and stayed on to become its faculty. It is here that Blalock's passion for newer surgical techniques and advanced experimental research took origin. He involved himself in the experimental animal lab of Vanderbilt and did several path-breaking works. Prominent of them was his work on shock research which saved thousands of lives during the war years and made him famous as a medical researcher.

During World War I and subsequent conflicts, a large number of soldiers died due to horrifying trauma, ruthless gunshot, and helpless blood loss. In Europe and America, the doctors commonly believed that such patients went to shock and their blood pressure dropped due to the presence of biochemical toxins and pathogens in their blood. It is called Crush Syndrome. When Blalock started his work, he had a different hypothesis. He believed and later proved by detailed research that "the cause of traumatic and hemorrhagic shock was due to blood loss externally as well as into the extravascular space". In this third space, between intravascular and intracellular space, fluid loss was the main culprit in such patients. He proved that giving blood or plasma serum to such patients in sufficient quantities would reverse the downward spiral of shock and save life.

Blalock's experimental work was validated and applied widely on the trauma patients, particularly on the war-injured soldiers. Thousands of lives were saved by his useful work. Blalock received praise and recognition because of his work which later became instrumental in getting him a prestigious offer from another hospital.

With the increasing burden of academic and surgical responsibility at Vanderbilt, Blalock could not find enough time for his experimental lab. He was looking for a suitable assistant as a laboratory technician. But it was difficult to find a person who was competent, skillful as well as who was able to follow the technical instructions exactly the way Blalock showed. It was not helping that Blalock was sometimes volatile with over-expressive anger making the life of the people working with him miserable.

In January of 1930, Dr. Blalock was sitting in his chamber when a lean, young, ordinary-looking black man walked inside. He told Blalock that he had come for a position of technician at his animal experiment lab. After interviewing him, Blalock found he had no former experience in laboratory or research work. However, the way he answered Blalock's questions stirred him in a significant way. Blalock took a chance and hired the man. Unbeknownst to him, this relationship would grow to become one of the most fruitful in his entire career and they would remain together till the day Blalock passed away in 1964. The two men developed a lifelong collaboration in the laboratory and in the training of surgical residents. The black lab assistant's name was Vivien Thomas.

***

In 1910, Vivien Theodore Thomas was born in New Iberia, Louisiana. He was the son of Mary and William Maceo Thomas. His grandfather was a slave. His childhood was spent in Nashville where he attended Pearl High School. Vivien's father was a carpenter by profession. He would always insist that his children had to learn his skills along with the regular education procedure. Hence, Thomas had to work with his father for two-and-a-half hours regularly after school and five hours on Saturdays. By the age of sixteen, he was able to perform difficult carpentry tasks without taking the aid of any assistants. What is more, he would be given money by his father for his effort every weekend. This was like a morale booster for him.

Thomas was a diligent student and was always good at his studies. He nurtured the ambition of becoming a doctor after finishing his college. He knew his family finances were poor. Hence, he used to save money whenever possible from whatever work he did. But his plans were completely ruined when a financial disaster stuck the United States. The 1929 stock market crash and the great depression wiped out all his savings. He also lost his job. Penniless and broke, with no hope for a college degree, he could manage a job of carpentry at the Vanderbilt University in the summer of 1929.

One early event in life taught Thomas a great lesson which he would never ever forget. He was just out of high school and was working on the Fisk University maintenance crew to earn money for his college tuition. One morning, Thomas had to work on a floor fixing a piece of worn flooring in one of the faculty houses. In the afternoon, the foreman came to inspect. He looked at the work Thomas had done and told him it was terrible. He left the place telling him to redo the flooring all over again.

Feeling humiliated, Thomas worked nonstop that afternoon. By the time the foreman returned, he had laid the pieces so beautifully that nobody could tell it apart from the original. The foreman was satisfied with the work and left. A few days later, Thomas met him at another place. The foreman told him, "Thomas, you could have fixed that floor right in the first place." These words really entered into Vivien's mind. He knew from that moment that no matter what he did—big or small—he must do his best. It has to be so perfect that the assignment will never need to have a repeat or improvement job. In the field Thomas was going to enter, it was indeed a very crucial lesson.

The economy was not getting any better at that time and many people were becoming jobless. Thomas was again fired from his job in the fall. After his luck ran out completely, Thomas asked his friend for a job at any position. He was guided to Blalock for an interview for lab technician at Vanderbilt University hospital. After the meeting, Blalock asked Thomas to join his lab from the very next day.

On the very first day at work, Blalock was impressed with Thomas's skills. For anything, he would just need to be instructed once. No matter what it was—whether a surgery on canine models or a difficult physiological experiment—Thomas would remember it forever on getting proper instructions. In the lab, Thomas soaked up knowledge like a sponge and nobody had done that before. He was always curious about the medical experiments at the lab and would continuously bother Blalock by asking endless questions. Blalock somehow seemed happy to explain and demonstrate everything in detail to this enthusiastic boy with no college degree or any research experience. Within a few days, Thomas was setting up complex experiments, performing arterial punctures in dogs, and was administering different anesthesia.

Soon, Blalock got a glimpse of Vivien's other skill, his dexterous use of fingers on the canine experimental surgery. As a good craftsman would recognize another, Blalock knew he had discovered "a gem". Blalock let Thomas start surgeries on the dogs at the lab while he instructed in the university hospital. That was a great advantage for both. In the daytime, Thomas would take care of all the lab works and Blalock could freely concentrate on his clinical work. In the evening, both would be together. They would work till late at night recording data, exchanging viewpoints, and mostly discussing high-level science. This arrangement worked well for both of them. Blalock got an expert assistant and Thomas a job.

For Thomas, there was another peculiar problem. At that time, black individuals were not allowed to hold technical positions at Vanderbilt University. Thomas had not even attended college. Blalock however found a way out. Thomas was classified and paid as a janitor. This arrangement continued despite the fact that by the mid-1930s, he was doing the work equivalent to a postdoctoral researcher in the lab.

The partnership forged by Blalock and Thomas was unique in medical history. Blalock had a style reminiscent of "southern aristocracy" and Thomas, the grandson of a slave as well as a black carpenter's apprentice, was "down-to-earth and straightforward". But in the lab, both shared a bond free from their social backgrounds. While Blalock would formulate hypotheses and questions of medical problems and research theories, it was Thomas who was hands-on and practical. Ever a craftsman, Thomas would find a way out for the most difficult of childhood heart defects. Thomas often worked up to sixteen hours a day in the experimental laboratory for a salary that was barely enough for him. This showed his passion for his job. Thomas had family obligations to consider too. In December 1933, he had married a young woman from Macon, Georgia, named Clara Flanders. Soon they had two beautiful daughters—Olga Fay and Theodosia.

At their blacktopped workbench and animal operating tables, the two men worked together diligently. This led to a number of major breakthroughs of the century and saved thousands of lives. Thomas was so talented that he could become a "cardiac surgery pioneer" with only a high school degree. He discovered numerous innovative techniques for approaching pediatric heart defects in the experimental models before they could be applied in humans. He also mentored and taught two generations of America's premier heart surgeons in his time when he himself could not become one.

People at Vanderbilt University were perplexed at their relationship. Some would condescendingly say, "it was merely a relation of convenience". But a surprise waited for those people who thought Blalock and Thomas's partnership was temporary. Blalock's research and prodigious presentations in peer-reviewed journals made him famous in the medical field. In 1937, Blalock was presented with a prestigious offer of Chairmanship from the reputable Henry Ford Hospital at Detroit. With this offer, he would become the Surgeon-in-Chief. He was also offered the sole autonomy to run his department, hire people, and conduct research.

The offer was a huge career break for Blalock. But when Blalock talked about Thomas to the Detroit faculty, there was pin-drop silence among the members of Ford Hospital management. The hospital had a strict policy against hiring black individuals. Blalock was told that any other demand was welcome other than this. His answer was simply unique—he boldly declared that he and Thomas were a "package deal". He refused to join if he was unable to bring Thomas with him.

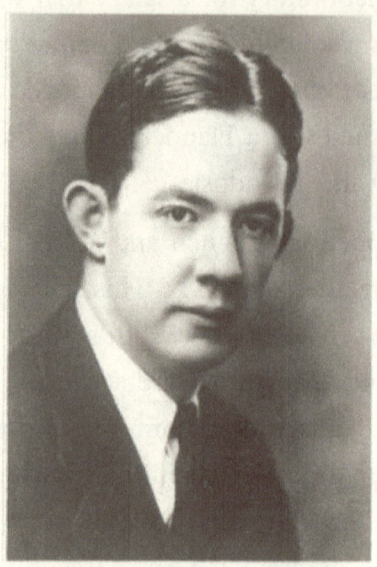

FIG: Alfred Blalock, a surgeon at the Johns Hopkins Hospital, operated on the world's first blue baby with a heart defect using a procedure known as the Blalock-Thomas-Taussig shunt.

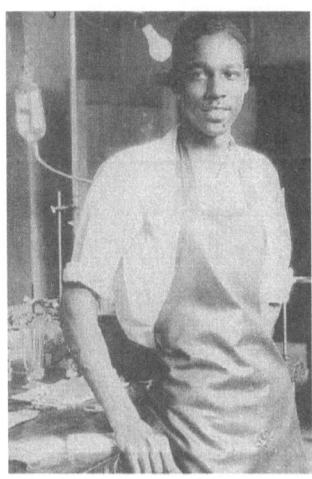

FIG: Vivien Thomas, the black young man who collaborated with Blalock to create BTT shunt surgery, the first-ever successful treatment of blue-baby heart disease.

A few years later, a much more prestigious, brand new offer was presented to Blalock in 1940. This was from Blalock's alma mater Johns Hopkins Hospital. He was offered to be the Surgeon-in-Chief and Director of the Surgery Department. This time, however, Vivien was not an issue. When Blalock asked him to move with him, Thomas took time for a decision. His family had settled down in Nashville. Besides, he knew nobody in Baltimore. After some thinking, he agreed to join Blalock. In 1941, at the age of forty-one years, Dr. Blalock joined as the Chief of the Department of Surgery at the Johns Hopkins Hospital and Thomas, ten years younger than him, was his chief lab assistant.

When Thomas arrived in Baltimore from Nashville, he found things were not what they had expected. **Hopkins was rigidly segregated just like the rest of Baltimore. The level of racism was more than what he had to endure in Nashville.** The houses in the race quarters were "cramped and gloomy". To make matters worse, the rentals and other costs of living in Baltimore were very high. His wife and children would often feel miserable in the new city which was bigger but not better for them. They would miss their extended family back at Nashville. There was hardly any opportunity for blacks in the formal sectors of

Baltimore in the 1940s. The only black employees at the institution were the janitors. Johns Hopkins' main entrance was forbidden for the blacks who had to use a side entrance to get into the institution. Washrooms were separate for black employees and were marked as "colored". When Thomas walked in the halls in his white lab coat, people would turn and look at him awkwardly. To avoid attention, Thomas began changing into his city clothes when he had to go to Blalock's office from the laboratory.

The workplace was also no less problematic for Thomas. When they had arrived, the experimental lab of Johns Hopkins was in a bad shape with years of neglect and underfunding. The Hunterian lab was like "a relic" with old instrument and control panels in a dusty old building. The technicians working had very average knowledge about the advanced experiments. They had practically no exposure to surgery of the animals for research purposes, a crucial part of Blalock's work.

Thomas, however, was at his quiet and determined best. He ordered his surgical supplies, cleaned and painted the lab meticulously, and then he painstakingly rebooted all the experimental instruments. Soon he put on his white coat and settled down to work. Before any time, Thomas put his life into the place. Working often late into the evening, he made the lab workable again.

Soon, Thomas and Blalock would be spending their useful and happy moments discussing or solving complex physiology of the vascular system and structural defects of the heart. This is what Thomas loved best. Whenever Blalock would throw any question or the practical challenge at him, he would find out an appropriate solution which many times surprised even Blalock, being the experienced clinician-researcher as he was.

***

While Blalock and Thomas were getting used to the life of Johns Hopkins, Dr. Helen Taussig was there all the time looking for a solution for her "blue-baby problem". After being refused by Gross at Boston, Taussig met

Blalock and pitched him the idea. Taussig told Blalock the problem she was having at hand. She also elaborated to him her theory of increasing the circulation of lungs by putting up an "artificial man-made shunt" from the systemic circulation into the artery supplying lungs.

Taussig finally got an opportunity to ask Blalock if he would be able to create the shunt for her to give her "blue babies" a chance to life. Blalock gave this idea a careful thought. Unlike Dr. Gross, he did not turn this proposal down right away. But he told Taussig that he did need some time to think about it. Technically speaking, such a shunt was surely possible, he told this to her. But he even said that he would prefer to test it first on an animal model.

When Blalock raised the problem in their usual evening chat, Thomas realized immediately that the answer lay in a procedure they had perfected for a different purpose in their Vanderbilt work. The intention then was to increase blood circulation to the lungs and create pulmonary arterial hypertension. For this, they had discussed about joining of the subclavian artery, the systemic artery supplying to arms, to the pulmonary artery. The Vanderbilt experiment had failed earlier, not giving the desired results they expected at that time. But both agreed that the same model might work in Taussig's problem.

Blalock and Thomas hoped that this increased blood flow to the lungs would help increase the general level of oxygen in the systemic blood. This kind of "plumbing job" by transferring blood from one circulation to another would not completely repair the defect. But it could work as well since the basic physiologic need was met. However, they needed to test the hypothesis in animal models to see if it worked before they could operate on any human babies. Blalock gave Thomas the responsibility of first creating a blue-baby-like condition in a dog, and then correcting the condition by means of the subclavian-to-pulmonary artery anastomosis.

In the meantime, problems for Thomas were getting worse at the "personal front". His household expenses were shooting up and rentals had crossed his budget and savings. Soon he would have to spend on the schooling of his daughters. To cover his expenses, he would do part-time jobs in the evening whenever he got spare time. Some of these evenings were spent at Blalock's home serving drinks to his guests. Awkwardly, many of the guests were the surgical trainees who at daytime would be learning experimental surgery under him.

Thomas's wife and children felt isolated missing the support system of their extended family at Nashville. In Baltimore, the neighborhoods were of migrant populations with very less personal interaction. The colored people had no social standings in the city. Many times, Thomas would think of going back to his old place with his family. It hurt him even more when suddenly one day he came to discover that his salary and rank at Johns Hopkins was the "same as that of the janitors". Finally, he discussed his problems with Blalock. Blalock understood his difficulties and was sympathetic toward him. His intervention with the Hopkins administration led to a reasonable increase in salary for Thomas so that he could concentrate on his work properly. This gave some relief to Thomas' troubled finances.

But no matter what happened outside and in his personal life, Thomas was always a perfectionist in the lab. He maintained unwavering accuracy in each of his surgeries or lab data logbooks. Once Thomas was inside the experimental lab with his gloves on, he would be concentrating purely on the work at hand. **Steady and quick, his fingers would move like that of a musician's on a piano or a ballet dancer's feet on the floor.** Undoubtedly, he was amongst the finest surgeons of the world. The only pitiable thing was that he was not licensed to practice in medicine. One can only speculate what he would have achieved if he were born in some other era.

Once while Blalock was away, Thomas created a prototype of a cardiac defect repair by operating on a dog. When Blalock came back, Thomas showed him the subject. Blalock took his time putting up his gloves and feeling the delicate "cuts and stitches" around the chambers of the heart. Blalock kept touching the specimen but could not find a single defect or irregularity on the entire surface. If somebody did not tell, one would not know that a surgery has been done at the site. While moving his fingers, Blalock suddenly became silent. Thomas was surprised and came closer.

"You have done this, Vivien?" Blalock asked grimly.

Thomas just nodded.

Blalock looked again at the masterpiece of work and said smilingly, "It looks like something the Lord made!"

Blalock was alluding to God's creation and comparing to Thomas'. That was the most amazing thing a southern white physician could have ever complimented a black man with, who neither entered into a college nor had any formal training in the field of cardiology.

Blalock was not the only surgeon who would marvel at the nimble fingers and dexterous hands of Thomas. All the surgical trainees of Johns Hopkins would get the opportunity to do so too. Some of the trainees were good while some others were average. Many of them would go on to graduate and become famous cardiac surgeons in their own capacity. Vivien would always teach each of them with utmost affection and patience, never judging any of them in the process. He would become a legend and an important part of Johns Hopkins folklore for years to come. "He never could become a doctor or operate on any person in his life, but he created dozens of highly skilled surgeons who after being trained by him went on to be famous surgeons in their own right".

One of the doctors trained by Vivien was the legendary cardiac surgeon from Texas Heart and was the first surgeon to implant an artificial heart; his name was Dr. Denton Cooley. He was also present in the operation theater during the famous blue-baby surgery of Dr. Blalock, the first such case ever in the world. Cooley was a great admirer of Thomas. "That's what I took from Vivien," he once said, "simplicity. There wasn't a false move, not a wasted motion, when he operated."

That day when Blalock left after discussing Taussig's problem, Thomas sat alone in the lab wondering how to replicate the blue-baby defect in dogs. Before proceeding for the real surgery, two important questions were needed to be answered. Would the Vanderbilt procedure relieve cyanosis in the babies? And most importantly, would delicate babies survive the effects of the procedure? It was known to Thomas that the systemic arteries had the blood flowing at a much higher pressure and velocity compared to pulmonary arteries. It was open to conjecture what would happen when the two systems were connected by a shunt.

Thomas knew it was one of the most important assignments ever handled by him. It would mean life or death to thousands of blue babies who would be operated depending on the results of this lab work. Thomas worked hard on the subject failing many times. Finally, after almost two years of laboratory work involving two hundred dogs, he was able to achieve the desired result.

One day, when Blalock came to the lab from the hospital, Thomas pointed his fingers toward a dog on the operating table. Blalock took a close look and was stunned. Thomas had created an "exact model" like the blue babies they wanted. Moreover, he had constructed an end-to-side connection between the subclavian artery and the pulmonary artery. And it worked too! With an abundance of oxygen pushed through the pulmonary artery, finally the systemic circulation began getting oxygenated blood. Blalock was overjoyed seeing Thomas's perfect surgical work. It worked appropriately in dogs; the time had come to test it for the first time on a blue baby.

***

When Blalock told Taussig about their readiness for the surgery, she invited Blalock to her pediatric ward. Together, Taussig and Blalock went to examine a baby. Blalock picked up the medical note hanging from the bed to look at the name. The baby's name was Eileen Saxon. About fifteen months old, she looked "desperately ill' and was being kept alive in an oxygen tent. Moreover, she was severely underweight, weighing only about five kilograms. Blalock noticed her lips and fingers. These were deep blue, and her skin was pale.

The child, Eileen Saxon, was born prematurely on August 3, 1943, at Johns Hopkins. Though the doctors detected a "heart murmur" upon listening with the stethoscope, not much was done about it. After a few months, the doctors noticed that Eileen's blood was not getting enough oxygen. She became cyanotic. Her symptoms worsened and she would become severely breathless, often losing consciousness. She had repeated admission into the hospital. Finally, she was admitted to the Harriet Lane Home at Hopkins on June 25, 1944, where the pediatric division was maintained and headed by physician Helen Taussig. By then, Eileen had badly lost weight and was looking malnourished and cyanotic pale.

It was definitely not a promising case and to top it all it was the very first such surgery in the world. Dr. Blalock's assistant Longmire was also disturbed seeing Eileen's condition. He felt the baby was "not fit for surgery at this stage". Blalock's anesthetists also frantically tried to avoid the surgery, and most of them felt that certain death was inevitable on the operating table. The Chief of Anesthesiology, Dr. Austin Lamont, actually declined the invitation, believing that the risk was too high and that induction itself could be fatal.

Blalock, however, stood his ground and the date for surgery was fixed. Hence, seeing no other option, Lamont somewhat reluctantly assigned Dr. Merel Harmel—his junior associate—to the task. Eileen was wheeled into the operation theater which was Room No. 706 in the early morning hours of Wednesday, November 29, 1944.

The operating theater was on the seventh floor of the building. It was a spacious room with two large windows providing ample amount of light. As baby Eileen was laid on the operating table, Blalock could finally see how "frail" she was. Her body was barely assessable under the surgical drapes. After anesthesia was administered, Blalock started the surgery. Assisting him were Chief Surgical Resident William Longmire and Nurse Charlotte Mitchell. A surgical intern Denton Cooley was at the other end giving saline and following small instructions. Cooley had recently joined under Blalock. He would afterward become one of the world's most premier cardiac surgeons. Standing beside the surgical team was Pediatric Cardiologist Helen Taussig. However, the person Blalock wanted most beside him was Thomas. He called out for him. Soon Thomas joined the operation theater and was standing just behind Blalock on a step stool, overlooking from above his shoulders. A little away from all of them, there was a small observation gallery where some doctors and staff of the hospital were eagerly watching what was going to unfold.

Blalock put an incision on the tiny chest of baby Eileen. The incision was an anterolateral part of the chest in the third intercostal space. Soon the second and third costal cartilages were divided to gain access into the chest. Blalock then dissected through the highly vascular mediastinum to isolate the left pulmonary artery. It was more difficult than what Blalock had imagined or practiced at Thomas's lab. Eileen's blood vessels were not even "half the size of those in the experimental animals" used to develop the procedure. When Blalock cut through, the blood oozed out thick and dark just as was the characteristic of cyanotic babies. Blalock first exposed the pulmonary artery, then the subclavian artery—the two tiny 'pipes' now needed to be connected. It was the most difficult part of the whole procedure. They had to move fast knowing well that Eileen had limited energy to tolerate a lengthy surgical procedure.

Blalock depended a lot on the experience of Thomas who had done the surgery many more times and knew each step by heart. Often during the surgery, Blalock would ask in a low tone without turning around, "Is this length of artery good enough?" "Is the incision long enough?" Thomas would answer from behind mostly agreeing and reassuring and sometimes even correcting. The back-and-forth exchange of sharp and short words would go on. "The two minds were so well connected that it was like two brains working with a single pair of hands".

The arteries of Eileen were so tiny that the edges would be impossible to suture with the help of normal surgical instruments. When Blalock was suturing the inner linings of vessels meticulously, he needed very small and fine instruments and needles. Since none was available in the market, those needles had been specially crafted by Thomas earlier during his experiments. Thomas had cut, bent and polished the needles to use in the small barely visible arteries. He also created many other instruments for clamping and pulling out vascular structures from the thoracic cage of the child while operating for better visualization and accuracy. It made the job a lot easier for Blalock. **With so little margin of error in a tiny underweight baby with cyanotic heart disease, these instruments created by Thomas would often be the major difference between success and disaster during the surgery.**

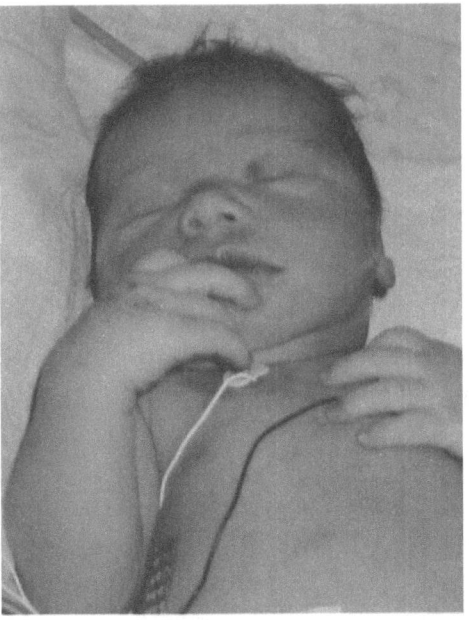

Fig: A Blue Baby with cyanosis

Blalock finally dissected out and freed the subclavian artery. Next, he cut into the pulmonary artery. He needed to make a small opening into which he would sew the divided subclavian artery. As Blalock made an incision in the pulmonary artery, he asked for Thomas' opinion to check if the incision was long enough or not. Thomas said that it would be fine. Blalock started a suture to delicately connect the two ends. Before he could proceed, he heard Thomas's voice and stopped. "It is in the wrong direction," Thomas quietly told him. Blalock immediately corrected himself to go in the opposite direction.

Finally, the anastomosis was made; the end of the shortened subclavian artery was connected with fine black silk sutures to the side of the pulmonary artery. The next step was to open the clamps which had held back the blood on both sides. The moment for which Blalock and Thomas had been preparing for more than two years had finally arrived. "In a few minutes, they would know if the baby's feeble lungs would tolerate the torrential blood from the systemic circulation of arm vessels; more importantly, if the excess flow would relieve the cyanosis or not".

When Blalock was satisfied that the surgery was complete and sutures were in place, he asked his assistant to help him remove the bulldog clamps that had stopped the blood flow during the operation. As soon as the clamp was removed, the blood started flowing across anastomosis shunting the systemic blood through the starving pulmonary artery into the lungs to be oxygenated. There was an immediate change in baby Eileen's vitals. When Blalock looked up "Eileen had turned pink"!

The next two cases of Fallot's cyanosis were soon operated. The second case was of a nine-year-old girl and the third child was a six-year-old boy. Both the children were showing classical symptoms of cyanosis. The boy was indeed so sick he could hardly walk a few steps unassisted. He was also severely wasted and malnourished. As it turned out, both cases were even better success. Finally, Blalock had proved to the world what was merely a theory in Taussig's mind. The first of blue babies had been operated on successfully. History had been made and will be remembered forever generation after generation.

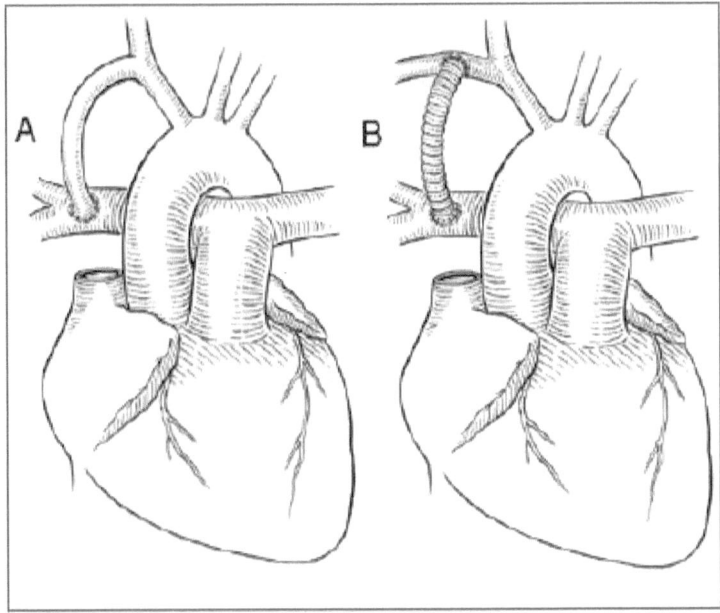

FIG: Blalock-Thomas-Taussig shunt surgery for treatment of cyanotic congenital heart disease of the blue-baby syndrome.

The surgery was like a miracle. Once, Blalock was operating on a blue baby. As soon as he finished the surgery and opened the clamp releasing blood from the subclavian to the pulmonary artery, the anesthetist cried loud from the other end excited. He called Blalock to take a look at the child's face. Blalock and Taussig moved to the head end from the bedside of the table. They were astonished at what they saw; "the baby had turned pink with healthy red lips". Within a few minutes, the baby recovered from anesthesia and asked to get out of the bed. It was a deeply moving moment for everybody present at the operation theater. **There could not be a better proof of the success of a procedure as immediate and as dramatic.**

For the next few days, many such cases were operated on. The children would get better faster than "anybody had ever anticipated". Nurses accustomed to tending critically ill children were often stunned to find babies who were previously desperate to run around and play happily. It was surprising to see the transformations.

In one of her case notes, Helen Taussig recorded, "His disposition has changed from that of a miserable whining child to a happy smiling boy."

Almost overnight Johns Hopkins and its 'Operating Room 706' became famous. Finally, after decades of turning the poor babies away, the doctors could face the parents of the blue babies and could tell them that there was indeed hope for them. The hospital was flooded with blue babies and their parents from all over the United States and abroad. The patients spilled over to other floors of the hospital. Blalock and his team worked almost round the clock for the whole of next year, barely taking a break except for the academic purpose of teaching the procedure to other hospital surgeons. **The results kept improving. It was the beginning of modern cardiac surgery.**

As the fame of surgery spread far across the world and a greater number of patients got admitted for surgery, Blalock became burdened with a huge workload. He leaned even more on Thomas for most of his clinical and lab work as well as records of data. Thomas never expressed any hardship of the job Blalock entrusted to him. He would often be seen running around the wards of Johns Hopkins with samples and notes. Afterward, he would go to the lab and keep working till late into the night. Besides Fallot's heart defect, there were many unsolved heart surgeries of children in those days. While Blalock did more surgeries at the hospital, Thomas did almost all the experimental surgeries in the lab starting from creating canine models to solving them.

Many distinguished surgeons and visitors would come to Johns Hopkins to see Blalock operating on blue babies. There was a viewing gallery in the operation theater, and they would stand and watch. Besides being party to one of the history-changing surgery, the visitors noticed a thing which was very strange. "It was Blalock's whine and also Thomas's presence giving advice that mystified the distinguished surgeons". Blalock would crib, shout and curse and be miserable at everybody during as well as after surgery being to the point of unreasonable. People would watch and would not understand why a famous surgeon such as Blalock was so hard on himself as well as the others.

Many individuals would say it was really difficult to go along with Blalock. Only Thomas knew what it would feel to become "a heart surgeon". Once somebody has been given over a baby to operate on its heart and cure it, he immediately became so unforgiving to mistakes. Measuring every length of step or every beat of work would become a habit to him. Gradually, those things become a heart doctor's second nature. The fear of messing up keeps their mind always "a little above anxiety and just a shade below paranoid". This trait is present in most of the cardiac specialists, though some are good at camouflaging it with outwardly friendly manners. Blalock was not one of them, though. He would be so straightforwardly upset about anything that went wrong in work or outside, even if it was his own mistake. **As he knew the consequences of even the tiniest of them, the burden of the life of those angelic kids would haunt him in every moment of his life.**

But Thomas would understand as only he could, as he felt the same sympathy and love for the dogs on whom he would operate to create models of heart problems of humans. Throughout his career at the experimental lab of Vanderbilt as well as Johns Hopkins, Vivien Thomas would not tolerate any lack of care or any sign of disrespect toward those animals. Many would die, often during the experimental heart surgery which was obvious. But to Thomas they were not mere objects of research; and this feeling bonded both the surgeons operating on hearts in a bond of unseen love which few could fathom. The Johns Hopkins people would often wonder what made a white southerner upper-class and a black carpenter's apprentice go along so well for thirty-four years.

To Thomas, whites would give racial comments and blacks would show resentment. He was hemmed poorly from both sides. But he would carry on with life never complaining once.

Blalock, with Thomas's help, collected all the data of surgeries and published the results of surgery. This was a landmark article that the medical community would sit up and take notice of. It was a "historical-first" surgery on a blue baby in the world. Besides the scientific people, a few press people got aware of the procedure and published articles in the mainstream press about this miraculous cure for blue babies. For the America struggling with bad news from the war, this came as a fresh new breeze. The news was widely reported making Blalock a national figure.

In 1945 in the month of May, a landmark article was published in the Journal of the American Medical Association written by Blalock and Taussig; it was titled "The Surgical Treatment of Malformations of the Heart in Which There is Pulmonary Stenosis or Pulmonary Atresia." It carried the elaborate details of the first three cases operated at Johns Hopkins—the cases which were brilliantly successful. It also described the lab research prior to surgery to test and validate the procedure. "Thomas' contributions to the procedure were overlooked, and his name did not appear on the manuscript".

In November of 1945, Blalock was invited by New York City's Harvey Society to give a lecture about the operation and the research that had made it possible. In the Harvey Lecture, Blalock acknowledged Taussig for her ideas about increasing blood flow to the lungs. Thomas, however, did not get any mention in the lecture from Blalock about his significant contribution.

Johns Hopkins became famous for cyanotic congenital heart surgery. The procedure itself was labeled as "Blalock and Taussig shunt"—named after two great physicians who solved the problem. But what the literary journals and media and public never mentioned was the third name—Vivien Thomas. The man who burned the midnight oil and contributed massively to the development of the actual technique and validation process but was never given any credit. When press and media came to take pictures of the team of doctors who were part of the successful surgery, everybody lined up including the assistant surgeons of Blalock, but not Thomas. It was an all-white picture of glory. In that era, black or colored people had only certain rights. Slavery was abolished by statute earlier, but equality eluded them for many more years.

In 1950, six years after Blalock had operated on the first blue baby in presence of Thomas, "Blue Baby No. 1000" was operated on successfully. It was a moment of glory for the Johns Hopkins and Dr. Blalock. A massive party was thrown to commemorate the occasion and honor Dr. Blalock and his team. Toasts were raised and champagnes were opened. Thomas did not get invited to attend the party. To commemorate the occasion, Johns Hopkins administration decided to honor Dr. Blalock by commissioning a portrait of him in the main lobby. The portrait by Yousuf Karsh came with "speeches and celebration" on a beautiful afternoon. Blalock was feted and praised wholeheartedly by his colleagues and the Director of the institute.

In 1949, *Life Magazine* brought out an article detailing the triumph of cyanotic heart surgery. It detailed the heroic perseverance of Dr. Taussig and the surgical genius of Dr. Blalock. It even mentioned Blalock's assistants in the surgery. Every step of the surgery, every turn in the difficult journey was chronicled beautifully. But Vivien's name was curiously missing from the pages. The magazine mentioned how Dr. Blalock had operated on a dog named Anna and seventy-five other dogs in painstaking research to achieve the final success.

Everybody at Hopkins knew that almost all the dog experiments were done by Thomas. The journalists did not want their readers to feel less heroic by being told that this was a black man's job. In those days, almost all the doctors in US hospitals were white males giving them an aura of benevolence and a savior. Black individual's sweat and blood mattered little and were insignificant. After all, even the blood for transfusion in blood banks those days was segregated. The blood bank carefully separated blood donated by whites from blood donated by blacks. Transfusing 'colored blood' to the white patients was considered as sin and was strictly prohibited. Even in the emergency cases, blacks were only occasionally allowed to receive a transfusion of 'white blood' when there was an urgency and no suitable 'colored blood' was available.

Blalock received accolades from the topmost universities in the USA for his epoch-making contribution to cardiac surgery. He spent a considerable part of his time on lectures and demonstrations to the aspiring surgeons eager to replicate his work. In 1947, Blalock was invited to Europe on a scientific tour. He reached London to have a royal reception. Blalock taught his surgical technique to the huge gatherings of British surgeons. At Guy's Hospital, he did ten of the surgeries with fair success. The press in Britain showered praise on the American surgeon. Toward the end of his stay, Taussig also joined him. Blalock shared the stage with Helen Taussig for a joint lecture to a packed hall at the British Medical Association. Their presentation was attended and acknowledged by the top surgeons of the UK with thunderous applause. Blalock and Taussig received recognition and fame across the Atlantic and it was enormous.

From England, Blalock traveled across Europe and then to several countries for his lecture tour. Wherever he went, Blalock and Taussig were given a huge reception and adulation for the unique surgery which benefited thousands of sick children across the globe.

During his lifespan, Dr. Blalock received a number of prestigious awards and honors. With his genius, he successfully received several honorary degrees from different American universities. His professional career also flourished. After doing thousands of successful surgeries, he was elected as Chairman of the Medical Board of The Johns Hopkins Hospital in the year 1955. He was declared both a Professor Emeritus of Surgery and a Surgeon-in-Chief Emeritus for The Johns Hopkins School of Medicine and the Johns Hopkins Hospital respectively while retiring in the month of July in 1964.

Dr. Blalock achieved the honor to be the member of forty-five national and international professional and honorary societies. These included the American Philosophical Society, the National Academy of Sciences, and the Royal Society of Medicine. He was invited to be a member of various prestigious committees such as the Subcommittee on Shock, the National Society for Medical Research, and the Board of Scientific Counselors. He was also an editor for seven journals including *Surgery, Archives of Surgery,* and *The American Surgeon.* Finally, Dr. Blalock received numerous national and international awards for his contributions to medicine. His most noteworthy awards include the René Leriche Award, the Matas Award, and the National Order of Merit from the Government of Cuba, the Modern Medicine Award for Distinguished Achievement, and the posthumous Henry Jacob Bigelow Medal in February of 1965.

The same was the case for Taussig as well. She too was successful in achieving international recognition and immense fame in her chosen field of pediatric cardiology. In the year 1960, she was named the honorary fellow of the American College of Cardiology. She received the "Gold Heart Award" in the year 1963. Again in the same year, she bagged Achievement Award from the American Association of University Women. Then in 1964, she was awarded Presidential Medal of Freedom by US President Lyndon Johnson. Finally in 1965, at the knowledgeable age of sixty-seven, she was able to become the first female President of the most esteemed cardiologic peer group in the United States: The American Heart Association.

Taussig was also able to bag a few other awards. These include "Chevalier Legion d'Honneur, Passano Award, Albert Lasker Award, the Herrick Award of the American Heart Association, the Howland Award of the American Pediatric Society, the Milton S. Eisenhower Award in 1976 from Johns Hopkins (the highest honor the University confers), and the highest civilian award, the Medal of Freedom in 1964."

Taussig was immensely elated that "her lifelong quest of providing some treatment to the blue babies had finally become successful". It was agreed by everyone as well as herself that she definitely deserved the recognitions showered on her. **Despite the many handicaps that** she had to painfully go through in her life—deafness, her mother's early demise, dyslexia, and to top it all, the sexist discrimination—she had been able to break all the barriers and reach great heights. For, a person whom Harvard mercilessly refused admission just for being a female had won every hurdle and acquired fame for herself as well as her institution Johns Hopkins.

But in the meantime, none of the honor, acclaim or admiration would wait for Thomas. For, all his hard work was the most crucial component of Taussig's hypothesis to be validated on bench before going into the operation theater. Without Thomas' years of labor, the first shunt surgery would have remained just that, a hypothesis only on paper. Thomas had harbored hope for becoming a doctor even in the years after the 1929 financial disaster and continued working at Vanderbilt. At Hopkins too for many years, he thought he could go back to college and pursue medicine. But finally, he had to give up. "In the face of pragmatism which prevailed over emotion and idealism". Thomas decided that it was the experimental lab that was going to be his choosing of profession. He continued to do this work, tried to excel in it, and also tried his best to be happy with what he had. He did not expect any medals or big honors as he knew that his desire would lead to a futile ending. Only a small recognition from the institute would suffice for him. Even a word from his dear partner in the endeavor, Blalock, would have meant a lot to his heart. But it never came: "neither from Johns Hopkins nor from Blalock". In the 1950s, it was not easy for the Americans to accept the contribution of a black for humanity in such a complex field as pediatric heart surgery.

Many years later, when Blalock died in the year 1964, a famous newspaper would report, following in obituary, ignoring any mention of Thomas who always stayed with him for more than three decades.

The news was printed as follows:

"BALTIMORE, September 15, 1964—Dr. Alfred Blalock, one of two physicians who developed the 'blue-baby operation' at the Johns Hopkins Hospital, died of cancer at the hospital today. He was 65 years old."

"Dr. Blalock was Surgeon-in-Chief of the hospital and Director of the Department of Surgery at the hospital's School of Medicine. He retired last July."

"The Georgia-born surgeon was 45 years old when, backed by years of difficult experiments, he joined with Dr. Helen B. Taussig, the hospital's Chief of the Children's Heart Clinic in 1944 to perform an operation that has since saved the lives of thousands of 'blue babies.'"

By this time, Thomas was utterly disheartened with the cold response for his years of hard and diligent labor. For some moments, even the thought of leaving Hopkins occurred to him. But he shook off the idea and continued working at Johns Hopkins lab. Above all, he loved his work and the boys he trained so meticulously. This was his world where he found comfort. He would not and could not leave it, with or without recognitions.

Blalock remained too busy in his work and research to notice the apparent discomfort raging inside Thomas's mind. Occasionally, Blalock would truthfully say to his residents about how much he would have loved Thomas to study medicine; but that was about all. Both Thomas and Blalock knew in their core that "it was just wishful thinking". **Time had passed by them, leaving two relatively old people in place of the two young hearts who started working in 1930 together.**

Over the next decade, Blalock continued to achieve further recognition as a great surgeon, mentor, and teacher. In the year 1948, in collaboration with Rollins Hanlon, a skilled cardiac surgeon, Blalock invented a technique for overcoming another congenital heart defect, the transposition of the great blood vessels of the heart. With his teaching as well as research, Alfred Blalock paved the way for a new generation of surgeons. As the Chief of Surgery at Hopkins, Blalock trained thirty-eight chief residents, nine chairmen of departments, ten division chiefs, and many others. His colleague and lifelong friend, Tinsley Harrison, the famous physician and editor-in-chief of "Harrison's Principles of Internal Medicine" spoke about Blalock's ability to teach brilliantly and said, "A teacher is an individual who has the capacity to influence the horizons of his pupils. Al (Alfred Blalock) has had that capacity all of his life." Blalock also had a prodigious research output in the form of numerous publications and books and scholarly articles across various journals. In 1955, Blalock became the Chairman of the Medical Board of The Johns Hopkins Hospital and held that position until his retirement in 1964. Upon retirement, Blalock held the title of Professor and Surgeon-in-Chief emeritus.

Life moved on usual till the year 1963 arrived, when Blalock suddenly fell ill. He had severe pain in his abdomen, which was found afterward to be urinary cancer. He underwent surgery which was not very encouraging in result. **"After years of mending hundreds of hearts and giving hope, this great surgeon had faced a personal challenge of the highest scale in his own life".**

Blalock's shining great professional career was about to end. He was in a wheelchair and was retired. Before Blalock would leave Johns Hopkins forever, he and Thomas met for the last time at the hospital. Both knew it was the end of their professional association spanning more than three decades. It was not easy though. Unspoken were the feelings and a relation, which was never defined—neither as superior-subordinate nor as friends. They exchanged some words reminiscing the old days. After a tour of the hospital with Thomas, Blalock walked out. Thomas looked on as the great surgeon moved away toward the sunset of his career. That was the last time the two would ever meet at the hospital. Three months later Blalock died on September 15, 1964. It was like the end of an era of genius. "By then the foundation of the heart surgery had been laid and well".

***

By the time Alfred Blalock retired and died in 1964, more than 2000 children had received the shunt at Johns Hopkins Hospital. Worldwide, more than 15,000 lives were saved by this procedure. There were also many versions of classical Blalock-Taussig shunt developed by different surgeons. One popular technique was called the "Modified Blalock-Taussig shunt method". Instead of using the complete subclavian artery itself, it adopted an artificial graft using a material called PTFE to achieve the anastomosis.

Another technique was called "The Central shunt" in which the anastomosis between the ascending aorta and the main pulmonary artery using a short PTFE conduit was achieved. In Potts shunt, which was developed as an alternate to CBTS in neonates, a connection is made between the descending aorta and left pulmonary artery. The objectives of these modifications were to regulate blood flow to the pulmonary artery and reduce the risk of closure of shunt prematurely.

In all these techniques, the basic principle of Blalock's surgery was intact. These surgeries were a great palliation providing relief to symptoms and helping in the growth of the children till the era of open-heart surgery arrived and the definitive intra-cardiac repair of tetralogy of Fallot was possible. From the day of the first surgery performed by Blalock, the field of pediatric heart surgery grew in variety and technique bringing in ever more children to a better life.

Over the next seven decades, there were staggering advances in virtually all aspects of pediatric cardiovascular medicine and surgery. These landmark achievements signaled the birth of the medical and surgical subspecialties of pediatric cardiology and congenital heart surgery. A lot of newer understandings came into the field of circulatory physiology and the abnormal morphology and functional consequences of structural congenital heart disease. These innovations saved lives and ultimately contribute to the mission of maximizing longevity. **Along with increased lifespan, the children living with congenital heart disease have had enormous improvement in the quality of life.**

***

"Roshan, stop!" I heard an anxious voice from behind the doors. I was about to enter the pediatric ward of the cardiac wing of our hospital.

Before I could make myself away, I was dashed in by a four-year-old child, running full steam ahead.

Before I could say anything, Roshan had already moved to the next room. I could hear the joyful excitement and exchange of words by the group of children in the other room.

Unless someone is told beforehand, a new visitor would mistake the place as a play school. However, this is the pediatric cardiac ward of our hospital. Many seriously ill babies, toddlers and school going age children with heart defects can be found at this place at most of the times. Some would be waiting for their turn to have heart surgery. Others, on the recovery path post-surgery, with bandages and venous catheter lines strapped to their chest and arms.

Children being children, they would not remember most of the times that a serious surgical procedure was the reason for them being in the wards. Roshan was also one of them. He along with other kids would create a play-list out of medical materials like cotton sheets, medicine bottle caps and small dispensers to make a game of their liking.

"I am sorry." Roshan's mother came out to apologize. "He is so naughty."

"No problem. When is his surgery?" I asked her.

"Tomorrow morning." She replied.

At that time Roshan came back. He hung to his mother, hanging like on a branch of a tree, and looked at me with wide eyes.

"Hi, Roshan. How are you." I said waiving my hand.

"I have a hole in the heart." Roshan said with disarming honesty looking at me.

"How do you know?" I Asked.

"Mummy was talking with 'the doctor aunty' that day". Roshan said in a matter-of-fact manner. He must have overheard the conversation a number of times.

"No problem. Tomorrow we will 'seal that hole'. There will be no more leak." I smiled and spoke.

"Will he be OK, doctor?" Roshan's mother asked, almost pleading.

"Of course. He will be absolutely fine after surgery."

My words had a convincing ring in them. I could see Roshan's mother feeling relieved. I could be so emphatic in my answer, which I knew was true. The confidence of modern pediatric heart surgery has been achieved by years of struggles, sacrifice and life risk to children suffering from congenital heart disease.

Today, heart surgery of children is significantly safe and successful. It is, thanks to the pioneers who toiled day and night to bring pediatric cardiology to a level which was only a dream few decades back.

A heart surgery on children in India has a success rate of more than ninety five percent. Babies with heart defect from many countries like Bangladesh, Pakistan, Nigeria, Ethiopia, Afghanistan come every year to india for the complex surgeries and go back with a successful result.

In the pediatric medical ward, it was time for medicines for the children. The nurse in charge bought in the medicine roller-tray. She reached out to each bedside, carefully took out medication for each child. Roshan sitting on his bed, lined with railings and saline stand, eagerly extended his hand to take the medicine.

"My mother says I will get to play with my friends at home if I take medicines regularly and get well soon." He told everyone.

I was getting a call from my resident from the other wing of the hospital. I squeezed Roshan's arms and moved on. From a distance I saw him waiving an enthusiastic "bye."

I could sleep comfortably that night, knowing for sure, Roshan will be smiling happily day after surgery, being cured of the heart defect which he was carrying since birth.

***

Pediatric heart surgery would not have grown as fast as it has without the boost by the "blue baby surgery" and the publicity it gave to the nascent field. After all, the heart was and continue to be one of the last frontiers of surgical science. All the other organs except the heart were by then amenable to somewhat appropriate surgical treatment. Soon after Blalock's work, the cardiac surgeons felt moved to solve many complex problems of the heart.

In the initial phase, what was achieved in the babies' hearts was just palliative surgery; that is, to remove the patent duct of arteriosus by ligation or creating a shunt like that of Blalock's. All this was done outside the heart itself, though it was very close to it and vessels were surrounding it.

Soon, the time came to surpass all this and go beyond. Cardiac surgeons were very eager to operate on other problems of the heart by reaching inside. They wanted to achieve the corrective surgery known as "total intra-cardiac repair". The difficulty lay in the fact that the heart, being a moving organ, was difficult to approach. One of the techniques which came up in the 1950s would help the surgeons to achieve their goal in a flawless manner. It was the "use of the heart-lung machine to achieve cardiopulmonary bypass".

Before bypass surgery was established, Dr. F. John Lewis performed the first intra-cardiac surgical procedure in the year 1952 when he repaired an atrial septal defect by using "moderate hypothermia and the caval inflow occlusion technique". The advent of the heart-lung machine in the mid-1950s marked a new era in the history of cardiac surgery. In 1953, after almost a lifetime of strenuous effort, John Gibbon performed the first open-heart procedure by using the heart-lung machine that he had developed, closing an ASD—a defect in which the upper two chambers of the heart called atrium are unnaturally connected by a hole. This was immediately followed by the repair of several moderately complex CHD diagnoses such as tetralogy of Fallot and complete atrioventricular septal defect. These surgeries were done by using a different method of cardiopulmonary bypass, "the cross-circulation technique" that was pioneered by Dr. C. Walton Lillehei.

John Kirklin from the Mayo Clinic accompanied by Richard Jones, who was a reputable engineer, paid a visit to Gibbon's Laboratory to elaborately study his heart-lung machine. Kirklin came back to improve Gibbon's screen oxygenator. The new device was much simpler to operate and had a comparatively lesser number of parts. This was named the "Mayo-Gibbon pump oxygenator". In the early months of 1955, Kirklin with the aid of this machine inaugurated the outstanding accomplishments in the Mayo Clinic Group's cardiac surgery.

Since the heart-lung machine could take over the function of the heart as a pump and lungs as the exchange of oxygen by the machine, surgeons had the advantage of getting a bloodless field and a fair amount of time to work and repair the cardiac defects properly. The very first patient was a child with a ventricular septal defect, " a hole between two lower chambers of heart". Afterward, many more children were operated on with the assistance of a heart-lung machine and the outcome showed fair results. Though hypothermia and cross-circulation technique briefly gained importance as competing techniques of attaining cardiopulmonary bypass during open-heart surgery, the heart-lung machine remained and continues today as the most important tool for cardiac surgery. In the meantime, Richard DeWall at the University of Minnesota developed a very simple, easy-to-assemble and to use bubble oxygenator. This discovery made use of the heart-lung machine more universal all across at several centers. Many more surgeons took up open-heart surgery and operated on congenital heart defects.

What also significantly helped the growth of pediatric cardiac surgery was the development in the field of diagnostics imaging in cardiology. Rapid improvement in ultrasonic imaging of the heart known as echocardiogram helped surgeons delineate the exact structural defects in hearts before the babies were taken to operation theater. The initial use of ultrasonic research was the use of high-frequency sound waves to find German submarines during the war times which soon found use in delineating structures underneath human skin in the abdomen and chest. Transesophageal echo was another technique where a small ultrasonic probe attached to an endoscope was put inside the food pipe. This technique was able to give much superior and life-like images of cardiac structures. Used intra-operatively, it helped to avoid many mistakes done on the table blindly which caused mortality or redoing surgery in earlier decades.

Later, cardiac MRI scanning and excellent multi-team approach in the form of dedicated cardiac nursing, nutritionist, physiotherapy, and rehabilitation specialists would provide a great support in improvement of the final outcome. Mortality rate of many congenital heart defects dropped dramatically from 70–80% to 5–10 % over just a period of a few decades. A large number of these children were able to have an almost normal life and were able to go to college, take up jobs, marry and raise kids. "If a baby had the misfortune to be born with congenital heart defects, of all the times in millennia, this was the luckiest time to be".

When open-heart surgery started in the 1950s and 1960s, the average age of the children during surgery was seven to nine years. The prevailing impression was that open-heart operations were poorly tolerated by the very young. The early cases of surgery in young babies one–three years old by the cross-circulation experience and other sporadic attempts at open-heart repair were found to have poor results and higher mortality. Surgeons, therefore, were apprehensive of operating on young babies with heart defects. Symptomatic neonates and infants were first subjected to palliative procedures, while intra-cardiac repair was delayed until the ages of five to seven years. This therapeutic policy presented serious disadvantages, though. Not only did it mandate two major surgeries on the child, but also the palliative surgeries often led to many "iatrogenic complications". Besides, the parents were burdened with the emotional burden of living with a threat of another operation as well increased cost of two operations.

In the late sixties and early seventies, Horiuchi et al. and Hikasa et al. in Japan, as well as Barratt-Boyes et al. in New Zealand, were successful in obtaining good results just with primary repair in the infants. The conclusion drawn was it is extremely useful for the baby to have a single curative surgery at an early stage of life. However, the skills and mechanical support needed for putting the tiny hearts under the operative lens were what daunted most surgeons. This extremely enthusiastic and encouraging approach was moved to a logical consensus level by an extraordinarily diligent doctor from Boston Children's Hospital, Massachusetts. This Harvard doctor with his skilled team was able to prove by a large group analysis that it is not only feasible but hugely beneficial to operate directly as intra-cardiac repair in neonates. He led the way to show that the best way to solve congenital heart puzzles was to "attack the problem at the very earliest" by not allowing the complications that cropped up by early palliation followed by delayed total repair. The name of this foresighted doctor was Aldo Castañeda.

Castañeda and his team at the Boston Children's Hospitals literally changed the whole outlook of congenital heart surgery to bring it to the present scenario. **After Blalock's work, Castañeda's is probably the most thought-provoking in the field of pediatric cardiac surgery.** Amongst the most difficult and challenging of his works was his study on babies with a heart defect called transposition of great arteries (TGA). Castañeda, who arrived from the impoverished Central American country Guatemala with a basic medical degree to the USA, has an enthralling life story that is as stunning as his remarkable achievement in the field of congenital heart surgery.

***

In a normal heart, the blood circulates in two series of flows. Oxygen-depleted blood, which is blue in color, is pumped from the right side of the heart to the lungs, through the pulmonary artery; on reaching the lungs it is oxygenated. The oxygen-rich blood, which is red in color, then returns to the left side of the heart through the pulmonary veins. Then it is pumped to the rest of the body through the aorta including the heart muscle itself.

In TGA (transposition of the great arteries), however, the connection of the two major vessels, aorta and pulmonary artery, are reversed and connected wrongly to opposite chambers. The deoxygenated blood from the right heart is pumped immediately through the aorta. Then, bypassing the lungs altogether, it is circulated to the body and the heart itself. In the meantime, the left heart keeps on pumping oxygenated blood back into the lungs via the pulmonary artery. In effect, two separate 'circular' circulatory systems are created parallel to each other, rather than the 'figure 8' circulation in series of a normal cardiopulmonary system.

If we imagine circulation like a house with its own water treatment system, in which the drinking water and cooking water after usage is sent by a plumbing system to the backyard, there this impure water goes into the treatment plant. But when the water comes out of the treatment plant, it is completely pure and is taken into the house for consumption or use by a pipe system.

However, in a TGA-like situation, the smoothly functional water-usage-purification-reuse circulation is broken by the mistaken switch of the plumbing. The household water after consumption comes out of the house through the drainage system. But instead of going into the treatment plant, it is re-circulated into the pipe going into house. On the other side, the water fed into the treatment plant comes out to go into the same treatment plant again by the faulty plumbing system. Thereby two separate circular systems are created. The home system is continuously being fed impure water and the treatment plant is for perpetuity cleaning already cleaned water. No wonder the system gets immediately wreaked! This explains why the babies with TGA (Transposition of Great Arteries) are severely symptomatic very early after birth, sometimes almost immediately in neonatal life.

The TGA is a condition of cyanotic heart disease second only to Fallot's tetralogy in the prevalence rate. It is considered a very complex deformity of the heart. Up to the 1970s, the diagnosis of d-TGA was the most dreaded analysis for the children. More than 95% of babies with TGA would die soon after birth. During that time, it remained one of the last of the unsolved cases of congenital heart disease along with the hypoplastic left heart.

Going into the historical background, it was Baillie in 1797 who gave the first morphological description of TGA. On the other hand, Farre in the year 1814, for the very first time used the term 'Transposition of Great Arteries'. Due to the massive anatomical deformity involved, it took almost one and a half centuries before a logical attempt to surgically cure TGA could be attempted by the doctors.

After the fifth decade of the twentieth century, a number of attempts were made by several centers to find a surgical solution to the TGA. The initial attempts were made to switch the atrial system so that the upper chambers of storage could be switched to connect to respective ventricles; hence the mismatch is corrected by the double mismatch. Since the atriums were receiving blood from the wrong systems, reversing the connection of the atrium to opposite ventricles would make the circulation correct. This method of correction of TGA was anatomically complex and afterward led to various complications like arrhythmias and valve leakage.

Afterward, it went through various modifications such as a venous switch, creation of baffle, atrial switch, and so on. Finally, it was discovered that the best surgical results were found by arterial switch surgery. This approach would attack the problem of TGA by its root cause. The two great arteries—aorta and pulmonary artery—which were connected to the wrong chambers were uprooted and connected by sewing to respective ventricles. This was a technically demanding surgery. This procedure was named as the "arterial switch operation" (ASO). A Brazilian surgeon of Lebanese origin named Adib Dominos

Jatene performed the first switch successfully and became the pioneer in this field; in 1975 at the University of Sao Paulo Heart Institute, Brazil. It was truly an anatomical correction in the form of an Arterial Switch Surgery.

Jatene's technique looked like the fair solution to the difficult problem that TGA was notorious for. But issues persisted even when the surgical technique was found. Initially, the children were taken for surgery after they had developed strength and weight. Many of the children would die of complications by the time they were considered suitable for surgery. Of the rest, a significant chunk also had by then developed various crucial complications in cardiopulmonary vascular systems. The heart would frequently become too muscular and hypertrophied. Several times it also happened that the collateral circulations would develop bypassing the original defects. Moreover, the pulmonary vascular system would be irreversibly affected making the long-term survival and quality of life less than that of a normal child. Many other issues like neurocognitive changes impacted the children as well. It is obvious that the only solution to the above problems is operating these as soon as possible, so that sequelae are not developed.

Many pioneering surgeons tried to bring the TGA heart surgeries to be carried about at one-two years of age through numerous attempts. But they had to helplessly face many technical difficulties like applying heart-lung machine to ultra-young underweight babies. The challenges were enormous, and the mortality rate was too high. Finally, the Boston team of doctors led by Dr. Aldo Castañeda would make the surgery of babies with these heart defects feasible. Castañeda operated on the babies literally "as soon as they were out of their mothers' wombs". The operation was performed on them at the tender age of as less as ten days. Just as it often happens in many outstanding discoveries that shatter the commonly held consensus belief to create a new paradigm, Castañeda too proved to the world that surgery on such tiny hearts was not only possible but extremely beneficial in the long run. This technique was called "neonatal complete repair of d-TGA".

***

Aldo Ricardo Castañeda Heuberger was born in Nervi, Italy, on July 17, 1930. His hometown was a seaside resort town near Genoa. He was born to Isabel Heuberger, originally from Nicaragua and Ricardo Castañeda Palacios from Guatemala. His parents were hardworking migrants. Early years of Castañeda's educational life were completed in Munich, Germany. It was during the time of World War II when his family was labeled as "aliens and foreign enemies" that they faced severe difficulties. As bombs dropped relentlessly on their locality, they lived in an underground bunker. At the age of fourteen, Castañeda survived in the basement of his family home while the structure above the ground was shattered to pieces by a bomb during an air raid. These events had a profound impact on Castañeda's life and thinking.

After the war ended, he studied in Switzerland for his college degree. In 1950, he was gripped with fear that World War III may happen in Europe due to the rivalry between the USA and Soviet Russia. He decided to leave Europe to go to his parents' country in South America. This may seem irrational today, but in his own words "as a young mind that has seen the devastations of war," this was a logical decision to him.

In 1951, Castañeda left Europe forever and reached Guatemala, Central America; he wanted to study medicine at the University of San Carlos. He excelled in his studies and graduated as the topper of his class. In 1958, he successfully bagged the Justo Rufino Barrios Prize for his academic excellence. During his time in Medical School, Castañeda conducted laboratory research on dogs according to a new technique for supporting the circulation with a bubble oxygenator and a motor pump. This was basically an "early version" of the heart-lung machine. This was a very recent concept in those days and hardly a few centers in the world had mastered such a technique. "It was an astounding achievement for a basic medical degree student in a country with virtually no research facility". Castañeda did his research without any mentor or practical exposure by merely reading from journals like *The New England Journal of Medicine* from his hospital's medical library.

Castañeda knew that the new technology on which he was working, was being studied and pioneered at the University of Minnesota. During the time after his internship, Castañeda applied to join the surgical research team in Minnesota and was accepted by Professor Owen H. Wangensteen. After his residency, Castañeda stayed on to be a faculty member at Minnesota. After some years of working there, the Boston Children's Hospital recruited him after a country-wide search for a new Chief of Pediatric Cardiac Surgery Program after hearing about his extraordinary abilities as a surgeon.

In Boston, Castañeda established one of the premier programs in pediatric cardiac surgery in the world. In collaboration with Alexander Nadas, the Cardiologist-in-Chief at the Boston Children's Hospital, he developed an integrated congenital cardiac program that included surgeons, cardiologists, cardiac nurses, anesthesiologists, radiologists, and cardiac pathologists to provide specialized care to children with congenital heart defects. This established Boston as the best among all the other children's heart centers in the world.

Castañeda's mission was to have the best possible results for all the children with heart disease on whom he personally operated. **He (Castañeda) felt with conviction that the babies with heart defect ought to have as good a life as a normal baby in all conceivable ways post-correction.** With this as his principal motto, Castañeda drove his team to cardiac research. The research done by them showed that deaths from complex congenital cardiac defects occurred mostly during the first few weeks of life. To reduce early deaths and to minimize secondary organ damages, including the heart, lungs, and central nervous system, this early surgical approach would also allow normal postnatal development, such as coronary angiogenesis, physiologic myocardial hyperplasia or hypertrophy, and pulmonary angiogenesis and alveolar genesis.

Based on this information, Castañeda was convinced that to achieve the near-perfect result in babies and to provide them "a normal life like any other person", they needed to be operated on within barely days of being born. This then gradually led to what later would become famous as the Castañeda doctrine: "Operate as soon post-natally as the patient needs it. Whenever possible, do corrective surgery, not palliative surgery. One operation is better than two (or more)." Aldo Castañeda by his groundbreaking work came to be known as the "father" of neonatal and first-year-of-life corrective congenital heart surgery.

The TGA surgery at age of one week just after birth is enormously difficult even today. Mostly, the babies are underweight weighing barely 700–900 gm, with the heart less than 30 grams of weight. They are also severely symptomatic and hypoxic. Giving them anesthesia is a tough challenge. In addition, Castañeda found that the heart-lung machines had never been used previously on such small babies. Post-surgery, there was also a question if the new left ventricle after the switch would be able to take the load of systemic circulations or fail. Surgeons feared the ventricle would break down without being primed for the load. All these problems needed to be addressed before TGA babies could be operated on at birth. Castañeda was well aware of the complex issues. He decided to go to the experimental lab before he stepped into the operation theater.

Castañeda initially took up some 2-kg-weight puppies and put them on cardiopulmonary bypass. In the beginning, the bypass was maintained for a few minutes and progressively increased the bypass time till they could achieve up to two hours. Afterward, the physiological and biochemical parameters of the puppies were checked to see if any permanent damage to the circulatory or organ system had occurred or not. The research convinced him that the effects of this two-hour period of an extracorporeal bypass on both the formed elements of blood and the lungs revealed only minor, transitory, and rapidly reversible changes that were well tolerated by these very young animals.

Armed with conviction from the lab research, Castañeda performed the first Arterial Switch Operation on January 2, 1983. He performed the operation on an eleven-day-old neonate with transposition of the great arteries and an intact ventricular septum.

Arterial switch operation (ASO) is one of the most complex neonatal operations requiring skill and precision to operate on a newborn heart weighing less than 20 grams. After the chest of the baby is opened and the heart exposed, the bypass is achieved by the heart-lung machine. Afterward, as a first step, the great arteries are divided. The next step performed on the heart is called "the LeCompte maneuver". In 1981, a technically important modification of surgically translocating the great vessels was described by LeCompte from Laennec Hospital, Paris, France, thereby avoiding the use of prosthetic conduit. Besides providing a better anatomical lie for the newly reconstructed aortic anastomosis and the coronary arteries, the method of right ventricular outflow tract reconstruction is greatly simplified by this during the ASO. The key to a successful ASO is the transfer of the coronary artery origins.

After the aorta is cross-clamped and divided, the sinus aorta surrounding the coronary ostia (the so-called coronary button) is excised. The boundary of the button is 1–2 mm of sinus aorta surrounding the coronary ostium. The commissure should be taken down when the ostium is adjacent to a commissure for ensuring that the button is large enough for coronary transfer. After the button excision, the proximal coronary is mobilized to allow the vessel to be implanted into the pulmonary root. After the coronary arteries are transferred, the great arteries are reconnected to the proper ventricle and any intra-cardiac communication is closed.

Castañeda's first neonatal ASO surgery was a success. For the next year, Castañeda with his team performed a series of such surgeries. In

1984, Castañeda et al. from the Boston Children's Hospital introduced to the world the concept of the neonatal arterial switch describing their experience with fourteen neonates. With this, there was an emphasis on the capability of the neonatal left ventricle for favorably handling the systemic circulation. "The end result left everyone with mouths agape".

After the procedure was complete, there remained the babies, who were suffering from TGA earlier, now almost on the verge of recovery with just a single curative surgery to be done. They were able to receive a near-normal anatomical heart with brilliant longevity. Today neonatal arterial switch remains the treatment of choice for TGA with remarkably low mortality; from a death rate of 95%, it came down to as low as 4%. This profound change was achieved by Castañeda and his team's relentless hard work on the tiny hearts of the one-week-old babies.

Although most surgeons would retire to a life of ease and comfort after such an illustrious career, Castañeda instead pursued his unwavering desire to better the lives of the children with congenital heart defects, particularly to those who were without access to care. In 1997, at the age of sixty-seven years, Castañeda returned to Guatemala where his father was born and he did his early medical studies. It was kind of his ancestral hometown and was close to his heart. Guatemala is basically a country of thirteen million inhabitants of mainly Mayan descent and twenty-three indigenous languages. During that time, there was no available surgical care for children with congenital heart defects in Guatemala.

In Guatemala City, the capital of Guatemala, he established a new program with the stated goals of providing clinical care for children with congenital heart defects, training the next generation of surgeons to continue the mission and conducting research. This center works as a referral center for children with heart disease and who were mostly referred from neighboring countries such as El Salvador, Nicaragua, Honduras, the Dominican Republic, Belize, and Haiti. This center has had a huge impact on the lives of countless children in the region who would otherwise not have survived to see their first birthdays.

Castañeda has received numerous honors and awards, including the Order of the Quetzal and the Order of Atanacio Tzul; both were presented to him by the Government of Guatemala. He has received the World Heart Foundation Humanitarian Award and has been named an honorary member of more than twenty professional societies around the world. He has received the Lifetime Achievement Award from the American College of Cardiology and has served as the seventy-fourth President of the American Association for Thoracic Surgery.

***

Alfred Blalock and Vivien's extraordinary relationship as well as their achievements at the Johns Hopkins in the backdrop of American socioeconomic history has been documented in the form of many stories, movies, and documentaries. In 2003, a Spark Media documentary *Partners of the Heart* premiered featuring the collaborations and lives of Blalock and Vivien Thomas at Vanderbilt and Johns Hopkins University. It was part of the PBS series *American Experience*. Written by Kalin and Lou Potter and directed by Andrea Kalin, the documentary *Partners of the Heart* successfully bagged Erik Barnouw Award presented by the Organization of American Historians and snatched the title for the Best History Documentary in the year 2004.

The 2004 HBO film *"Something the Lord Made"* was again about the Blalock–Thomas collaboration, which became the winner of three Emmy Awards—for Outstanding Cinematography for a Miniseries or Movie, Movie or a Special and Outstanding Made for Television Movie, and Outstanding Single-Camera Picture Editing for a Miniseries. In a very real-life manner, the relation of the two men of starkly opposite statuses, but who were equal in heart, is depicted in the movie. The script is developed on Katie McCabe's *Like Something the Lord Made* featuring in the *Washingtonian*. Alan Rickman played the role of Blalock and Mos Def played the role of Thomas. The film was produced by Robert Cort.

It was a fine day in the month of August 2019, when a tall and thin-built white man walked into the atrium of Johns Hopkins Children's Center. When the information receptionist looked up to him, he greeted her politely saying, "Hi! My name is Hugh Michael Edenburn. I was brought into Johns Hopkins 70 years back by my mother all the way from Iowa. I was labeled Blue Baby #44 by Dr. Taussig. I was operated by Dr. Blalock in May 1945."

The receptionist was too shocked to answer anything to Edenburn. The only thing she could utter was "Oh my God! You're *history!*"

She was right! The two-year-frail baby of the year 1945 had lived through life all the way. On that very day, he was 76 years old and was fit and healthy; he made all the doctors and staff at Hopkins thrilled. "After all, the story came back from where it all started".

Edenburn happily narrated his life's story to the hospital staff. He began the story from the day he arrived from Iowa with his mother as a two and half year baby in 1945 to try his luck with the then-new surgery. Dr. Taussig immediately logged Edenburn into her patient registry as "The Blue Baby #44". Dr. Blalock operated on him afterward. The operation was a tremendous success. Over the next six years, Edenburn had follow-up visits at the Johns Hopkins before his family moved to Worcester, Massachusetts.

Edenburn did well for many years except for a little breathing difficulty now and then which got worse with extra effort. Then, at the age of 18, events presented another challenge in front of him. While he was being treated at Yale for injuries from an automobile accident, doctors diagnosed him with subacute bacterial endocarditis, an infection which happens on the lining of the heart. After assessing the teenager's breathing difficulties and his medical history, the physicians recommended an updated tetralogy of Fallot repair.

After that Edenburn never had to look back. His entrepreneurial spirit led him first to build a startup office-cleaning venture and then, thanks to his brilliant talent for technology, his own computer business. His successful business work took him around the globe to various countries. He was also involved in a charity organization as Gift of Life Program in the Philippines which provides help in getting heart surgeries of children from poor families. He has paid back the 'gift of life' he got seventy years back in the compassionate hands of Dr. Blalock encouraged by Dr. Taussig and assisted by Thomas. His life, like many others operated on for various heart disorders, is a big *"Thank You"* to the team of Johns Hopkins and all the doctors in the world who never let themselves waver from the belief that they can find a cure for what was then an insurmountable problem.

These hardworking heart doctors never let anyone think for a moment that the word "impossible" ever existed for them. Like 'angels of heart' they would guard the children day and night thwarting any complication that came in the way. These doctors transformed the scene from "hopelessness to optimism", from "despair to success". From all the babies who got cured of heart defects and could not come back to say a heartfelt 'thanks', it was Edenburn who conveyed the message.

***

After Blalock walked away from the main hall of Hopkins Hospital leaving Thomas behind on that fateful day in 1964, just a few months before he died, Thomas just stopped for a moment. Then, he walked back to his workplace, the experimental research lab of Johns Hopkins. There he continued to work with the same focus and dedication as he did for the last twenty-five years. There was no publicity, no expectation of any great honor from either Johns Hopkins or from the academic scientific world. It was plain and simple hard work, away from the limelight. Now he had a team of young apprentices. Thomas made sure they were well-trained as lab technicians and got selected to be working in the biggest of heart centers all across the United States. His love for animals was always legendary. Even those dogs that had to be cut open and afterward needed to be killed would have his extraordinary care and love. "For him, they were his animals first and experimental subjects dedicated to humanity later. His kindness to the trainee doctors would be famous as ever".

People who worked with Thomas had the utmost respect for his "extraordinary work ethic, vision, intelligence, and skills in surgery". What was missing though, was the acknowledgment from the world about his contribution to cardiology. Nobody would know how he felt about that. Whatever little pain Thomas would "carry in his heart", he rarely shared with anybody. A few people close to him only understood his contributions and hard work. They were very sad that Thomas was not given the due recognition that all knew he deserved. **It looked as if this grandson of a slave and a black man with the "wizardry of experimental cardiac surgery" would move to his sunset just like that.**

But things changed with the passage of time and took a surprisingly positive turn. First, it came from the surgical trainees and their admiration and affection that Thomas valued the most. The early batches of surgical trainees were now famous and legendary in their own right. They were known as the 'Old Hands'—Henry Bahnson, Rollins Halon, Denton Cooley, David C. Sabiston jun and Mark Ravitch, to name a few. They had continued to maintain ties with their beloved mentor 'Mr. Thomas'. Whenever they were faced with a surgical challenge or even had to do a major complex cardiac surgery, they would call Thomas to seek advice. Year after year, the 'Old Hands' would take time out from their work to come back to Hunterian lab to meet Thomas.

In 1969, formally known as the Halsted residents, the 'Old Hands Club' unanimously voted for commissioning a portrait of Thomas and it was to be presented to Johns Hopkins institutions. Then finally on February 27, 1971, the portrait was unveiled in a ceremonial function in the presence of the President of American College of Surgeons, other 'Old Hands', and the Chief of Surgery of at Johns Hopkins. Thomas came there with his wife, Clara. A formal presentation ceremony was held at the Hopkins auditorium. For the very first time in thirty-one years, Thomas rose to thank the distinguished gathering. It was a rare experience for Thomas, who always had toiled behind the scenes all the years.

As Thomas stood at the center stage for the presentation ceremony, looking at the gathering of the most famous surgeons from United States; he said that he was feeling "quite humble, but at the same time, just a little bit proud."

It was a rich recognition from the cardiac surgery's hall of fame. Thomas, humble as always, would express his surprise at his portrait being painted and formally presented. It was the words of hospital President Dr. Russell Nelson that delivered the theme, "There are all sorts of degrees and diplomas and certificates, but nothing equals recognition by your peers."

Everyone present at the ceremony wondered where Vivien's portrait would hang. The astounded gathering gave a rousing welcome applause when Dr. Nelson stated, "We are going to hang your fine portrait with Professor Blalock. We think you 'hung' together, and you had better continue to 'hang together.'" **There could not be a better expression, a pair of genius incomplete without each other, finally getting the place they deserved.** Today, for any visitor to Johns Hopkins Hospital, it is a must to stand and watch the portraits of Blalock and Thomas hanging beside each other in the lobby of the Alfred Blalock Clinical Science building.

Five years later, on May 21, 1976, the recognition of Vivien Thomas's achievements was complete when Johns Hopkins awarded him an honorary doctorate and an appointment to the Medical School faculty. On April 16, 1976, Thomas received a letter from Steven Muller, the President of the Johns Hopkins University. This letter stated that the Board of Trustees had voted to award Thomas with an honorary degree at the One-Hundredth Commencement Ceremony. As the news spread throughout the university, "friends as well as strangers offered Thomas their congratulations".

The poster gallantly flashed the name *Vivien Theodore Thomas, Doctor of Laws* as it was unveiled and a thunderous applause filled the air with glee. Thomas received the scroll as he stood in his gold-and-sable academic robe, for the awarding of the degree. "The applause was so great that I felt very small," Thomas wrote later. This sage-like black man had not even a bit of bitterness in his heart that it took Johns Hopkins thirty-five years to give the degree, which was maybe longest ever for any of its students.

Not only does Thomas's legacy live on through the people he mentored, but his work has inspired the creation of many programs and awards. In 1993, the Congressional Black Caucus Foundation established the Vivien Thomas Scholarship for Medical Science and Research. Sponsored by GlaxoSmithKline, this scholarship is available to "meritorious but financially disadvantaged students" who are pursuing a degree in the medical sciences. The Council on Cardiovascular Surgery and Anesthesiology started the Vivien Thomas Young Investigator Award in 1996. Lastly, in 2004, Baltimore City Public School System created the Vivien T. Thomas Medical Arts Academy.

Finally, after decades of when it happened, the surgery Thomas created with his sweat and perseverance was officially recognized in the textbooks of medicine and research journals as Blalock–Thomas–Taussig shunt—finally adding his name to the two illustrious persons like just as it deserved to be.

In 2004, The Johns Hopkins University School of Medicine announced the establishment of the Vivien Thomas Fund for Diversity to increase the number of minorities in the academic medicine talent pool. The proposal described by the following announcement, "The memory of the African-American surgical technician is basically honored by this fund. It was Thomas, whose pivotal offerings sixty years ago to the advancement of the 'blue-baby operation', who paved the way for the era of heart surgery at Hopkins." Edward D Miller, M.D., Dean, and CEO of Johns Hopkins Medicine once said, "We can best honor Vivien Thomas by removing for others the economic and racial barriers that often stood in his way."

A young black person joined Johns Hopkins as a medical student in the year 1982. His name was Koco Eaton. He was Vivien Thomas' nephew. The day Koco walked the corridors of Johns Hopkins with his shining white lab coat, "heads turned toward him", but this time because he was Vivien Thomas' nephew and not because of his skin color. Thomas was very happy that his nephew could get the opportunity to serve mankind which was denied to him a generation earlier as he was not up to a certain color. Koco was trained by the same men who were trained by Thomas and were faculty now. Every morning when Koco would enter Johns Hopkins to attend medical lectures, it would be through the main entrance; and not the side passage that Thomas and the likes used in a reverse time lag.

And to Vivien Thomas, how much it mattered that a historical injustice had been corrected to some extent would never be known to anyone; as from his outer demeanor he would always remain the same—soft-spoken, hardworking; crafting ingenious solutions for tiny broken hearts. For him the world remained unaltered, only the clock had moved to a better time.

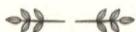

Thank you for picking up this book and going along the journey of compassionate and loving indivisuals lives spanning a century. If you like any of the stories, characters or chapters of this book please write to me on Facebook /instagram link @ lingaraj nath or mail me to drlrnath@gmail.com. Your valuable opinion will be appreciated and acknowledged by me.

– Author

ACKNOWLEDGMENT

I would like to thank Nyra Sen, Editor and Anamika Roy Choudhury, Manager of 24by7 publishing for their best support and guidance during the book creation process. You both have been very instrumental in transforming my book from an idea to a full manuscript.

Thanks to Chandrika Taleja for initiating me into Notion Press. Ever since that day, it had been a pleasant ride to the release of this book. Thanks to Ashwin S for creating the face and identity of my book in a beautiful manner by designing the cover image.

Thanks to Mangala Komarathfor performing surgery on the content and making it come to an even perfect shape.

Special thanks to Sarvesh S for being my partner, friend and publishing manager in the whole publishing process of my book. We were a great team!

Finally, I sincerely acknowledge my teachers, colleagues, fellow cardiologists, cardiac surgeons, and the dedicated nurses and cardiac technicians who have always inspired me in my work. I am ever indebted to my patients who have effortlessly put immense faith in my ability in every situation.

NOTES

Chapter 2: Angels of Heart

1. J Thorac Cardiovasc Surg. 2012 Feb; 143(2): 260–263.

   PMCID: PMC4128896 NIHMSID: NIHMS617784. PMID: 22248679

   Centennial Presidential Perspective: Dr. Alfred Blalock

   Claude A. Beaty, M.D.,1 Timothy J. George, M.D.,1 and John V. Conte, MD1

2. Pediatric Cardiology and Cardiovascular Surgery: 1950–2000

   Robert M. Freedom, James Lock, and J. Timothy Bricker

   Originally published, 22 Mar 2018 Circulation. 2000;102:Iv-58–Iv-68

3. Pediatric Cardiac Surgery: The Long View

   Marshall L. Jacobs

   Circulation. 2015;131:328–330

4. Thorac Cardiovasc Surg. 2010 Sep;58(6):318-9.

   Aldo Ricardo Castañeda, M.D., PhD: What Is He Really Like?

   R. van Praagh. Cardiac Registry, Children's Hospital, Boston, Massachusetts, United States

5. Ann Thorac Surg. 1997 Nov;64(5):1544-8.

   Early development of congenital heart surgery: open-heart procedures

6. Bhimji, Shabir. "Tetralogy of Fallot." Medscape

7. Blalock, Alfred, and Helen Taussig. "The Surgical Treatment of Malformations of the Heart in which there is Pulmonary Stenosis or Pulmonary Atresia." The Journal of the American Medical Association 128, no. 3 (1945): 189-202 62

8. Bonchek, Lawrence I., Albert Starr, Cecille O. Sutherland, and Victor D. Menashe. "Natural History of Tetralogy of Fallot in Infancy: Clinical Classification and Therapeutic Implications." Circulation 48 (1973): 392-397.

9. Brogan, Thomas V., and George M. Alifieris. "Has the time come to rename the BlalockTaussig shunt?." Pediatric Critical Care Medicine: A Journal Of The Society Of Critical Care Medicine And The World Federation Of Pediatric Intensive And Critical Care Societies 4, no. 4 (2003): 450-453.

10. Davis, Ronald L.F.. "Racial Etiquette: The Racial Customs and Rules of Racial Behavior in Jim Crow America." The History of Jim Crow.

11. Evans, William N.. "Tetralogy of Fallot and Étienne-Louis Arthur Fallot." Pediatric Cardiology 29 (2008): 637-640.

12. Evans, William N.. "Blalock-Taussig shunt: the social history of an eponym." Cardiology in the Young 19 (2009): 199-128.

13. Forde, Richard James. Jewish Women: A Comprehensive Historical Encyclopedia, s.v. "Helen Brooke Taussig.": Jewish Women's Archive.

14. Gale, Thomson. Encyclopedia of World Biography, 1 ed., s.v. "Taussig, Helen Brooke." Detroit: Gale, 1998.

15. Gee, Bob. Vivien Theodore Thomas. 1969. The Johns Hopkins Medical Archives, Baltimore. Accessed 21 Mar. 2012. 63 Greevy, James M.. "The Other Contributions of Alfred Blalock." Current Surgery 60, no. 2 (2003): 160-163

16. Harvey, W. Proctor. "A Conversation with Helen Taussig." Medical Times 106, no. 11 (1978): 28-44.

17. Hughes, Everett Cherrington. "Dilemmas and Contradictions of Status." The American Journal of Sociology 50, no. 5 (1945): 353-359.

18. Longmire, William P.. Alfred Blalock: his life and times. Washinton D.C.: Vanity Press, 1991.

19. Maloney, Thomas. EH.net Encyclopedia, s.v. "African Americans in the Twentieth Century." Economic History Association, 2002.

20. Oylu, Erdinc; Athanasiou, Thanos; Jarral, Omar A (May 2017). "Vivien Theodore Thomas (1910–1985): An African-American laboratory technician who went on to become an innovator in cardiac surgery". Journal of Medical Biography. 25 (2): 106–113.

21. Tex Heart Inst J. 2005; 32(4): 477-478. PMCID: PMC1351817.PMID: 16429890

In Search of Vivien Thomas

Damon M. Kennedy, DO

22. McCabe, Katie. "Like Something the Lord Made." The Washingtonian, August 1989, 108-111, 226-233.
23. Neill, Catherine A., and Edward B. Clark. "Tetralogy of Fallot: The First 300 Years." Texas Heart Institute Journal 21, no. 4 (1994): 272-279.
24. Parsons, Isabell Hunner. Alfred Blalock. 1945. The Johns Hopkins Medical Archives, Baltimore. Accessed 21 Mar. 2012.
25. Partners of the Heart. Dir. Andrea Kalin. Spark Media, 2003. DVD Schmoop Editorial Team. "Jim Crow." Shmoop: Homework Help, Teacher Resources, Test Prep.
26. Taussig, Helen. "A Conversation with Helen Taussig," interview by W. Proctor Harvey. 64 Medical Times 106, no. 11 (November 1978): 28-44.
27. Thomas, Vivien. "Mr. Vivien Thomas Discusses Dr. Alfred Blalock," interview by Peter D. Olch. Tape recording. National Library of Medicine Archives and Modern Manuscripts Oral Histories Collection. Baltimore, Maryland. April 20, 1967.
28. Thomas, Vivien T.. Partners of the heart: Vivien Thomas and his work with Alfred Blalock: an autobiography. Philadelphia: University of Pennsylvania Press, 1998.
29. Timmermans, Stefan. "A Black Technician and Blue Babies." Social Studies of Science 33, no. 197 (2003): 197-229.
30. Toledo-Pereyra, Luis H. "Alfred Blalock. Surgeon, Educator, and Pioneer in Shock and Cardiac Research. " Journal of Investigative Surgery 18, no. 4 (2005): 161-165.
31. Wooley, Charles F., and Pamela J. Miller. "William Osler, Maude Abbott, Paul Dudley White, and Helen Taussig: the origins of congenital heart disease in North America." The American Heart Hospital Journal 6, no. 1 (2008): 51-56.

32. Ann Pediatr Cardiol. 2015 May-Aug; 8(2): 122–128.

   PMCID: PMC4453180.PMID: 26085763

   Surgery for transposition of great arteries: A historical perspective

   Supreet P Marathe and Sachin Talwar1

Chapter 3: Turn the Clock Back

1. Curr Probl Cardiol. 2010 Feb; 35(2): 72–115.

   PMCID: PMC2864143. NIHMSID: NIHMS170650. PMID: 20109979

   Growing Epidemic of Coronary Heart Disease in Low- and Middle-Income Countries

   Thomas A. Gaziano, M.D., MSc,*† Asaf Bitton, M.D.,* Shuchi Anand, M.D.,* Shafika Abrahams-Gessel, MS,‡ and Adrianna Murphy†

2. Heart Views. 2017 Apr-Jun; 18(2): 68–74.

   PMCID: PMC5501035. PMID: 28706602

   Coronary Heart Disease: From Mummies to 21st Century

   Rachel Hajar, M.D.

3. Coronary artery disease

   Urbanization is a risk factor for CAD

   Irene Fernández-Ruiz

   Nature Reviews Cardiology volume 14, page252(2017)

4. Kaplan, H. et al. Coronary atherosclerosis in indigenous South American Tsimané: a cross-sectional cohort study. Lancet http://dx.doi.org/10.1016/S0140-6736(17)30752-3 (2017)

5. Anitschkow NN, Chatalov S (1913). „Über experimentelle Cholesterinsteatose und ihre Bedeutung für die Entstehung einiger pathologischer Prozesse". Zentralbl Allg Pathol. 24: 1–9.

6. J Thorac Dis. 2018 Mar; 10(3): 1960–1967.

   PMCID: PMC5906252. PMID: 29707352

   Fifty years of coronary artery bypass grafting

   Ludovic Melly,1,* Gianluca Torregrossa,⊠2,* Timothy Lee,2 Jean-Luc Jansens,1 and John D. Puskas

7. Dotter C, Judkins M (1 November 1964). "Transluminal treatment of arteriosclerotic obstruction. Description of a new technic and a preliminary report of its applications". Circulation. 30 (5): 654–70. doi:10.1161/01.CIR.30.5.654. PMID 14226164.

8. Front Cardiovasc Med. 2014; 1: 15.

   Published online 2014 Dec 29. PMCID: PMC4671350. PMID: 26664865

   Balloon Angioplasty – The Legacy of Andreas Grüntzig, M.D. (1939–1985)

   Matthias Barton,1,* Johannes Grüntzig,2 Marc Husmann,3 and Josef Rösch4

9. Sette P, Dorizzi RM, Azzini AM. Vascular access: an historical perspective from Sir William Harvey to the 1956 Nobel Prize to André F. Cournand, Werner Forssmann, and Dickinson W. Richards. J Vasc Access (2012) 13(2):137–44.10.5301/jva.5000018

10. Am Heart J. 1995 Jan;129(1):146-72.

    The history of interventional cardiology: cardiac catheterization, angioplasty, and related interventions

    R L Mueller 1, T A Sanborn

11. Grüntzig AR, Senning Å, Siegenthaler WE. Nonoperative dilatation of coronary-artery stenosis: percutaneous transluminal coronary angioplasty. N Engl J Med (1979) 301(2):61–8.10.1056/NEJM197907123010201

12. Hurst JW. The first coronary angioplasty as described by Andreas Gruentzig. Am J Cardiol (1986) 57(1):185–6.10.1016/0002-9149(86)90981-1

13. King SB., III The development of interventional cardiology. J Am Coll Cardiol (1998) 31(4 Suppl B):64B–88B.10.1016/S0735-1097(97)00558-5
14. King SB. As I knew him. Cardiology (1986) 73(4–5):192–3.
15. Hurst JW. Andreas Roland Gruentzig, M.D.: the teaching genius. Clin Cardiol (1986) 9(1):35–7.10.1002/clc.4960090109
16. King SB. Legends in Cardiology: Andreas Gruentzig, M.D. (1939-1985). (1985).
17. Nuncius. 2011;26(1):132-58.

    Voyaging in the vein: medical experimentation with heart catheters in the twentieth century

    Ramona Braun
18. Interventional Cardiology (S Rao, Section Editor) Published: 23 December 2015

    The History of Primary Angioplasty and Stenting for Acute Myocardial Infarction

19. Nathaniel R. Smilowitz & Frederick Feit

    Current Cardiology Reports volume 18, Article number: 5 (2016)
20. American Heart Journal. Volume 129, Issue 1, January 1995, Pages 146-172

    The history of interventional cardiology: Cardiac catheterization, angioplasty, and related interventions

    Richard L.MuellerMDTimothy A.SanbornM.

Chapter 4: A Gift From The Heart

1. Piller, Laurence William. The Cardiac Clinic, Groote Schuur Hospital 1951-1972. The Schrire Years. South Africa Published by comPress, 2000.
2. Heart of Capetown museum website

   Louis Washkansky: The brave man with the new heart
3. History of cardiac surgery

   M K Davies, A Hollman. BMJ Journals. HEART Volume 87, Issue 6.2002
4. Tex Heart Inst J. 2011; 38(5): 486–490.

   PMCID: PMC3231540.PMID: 22163121

   Cardiac Surgery: A Century of Progress; Allen B. Weisse, M.D.
5. S Afr Med J, "A human cardiac transplant: an interim report of a successful operation performed at Groote Schuur Hospital, Cape Town", Barnard CN, 1967 Dec 30; 41(48): 1271–74.
6. Cardiovasc J Afr. 2009 Feb; 20(1): 31–35. PMCID: PMC4200566. PMID: 19287813

   The first human heart transplant and further advances in cardiac transplantation at Groote Schuur Hospital and the University of Cape Town. Johan G Brink, MB ChB, FCS (SA) (Cardthor)
7. January 2002Volume 123, Issue 1, Pages 1–2

   Christiaan Neethling Barnard (1922-2001)

   Malek G. Massad, M.D.

   In Memoriam| Volume 123, ISSUE 1, P1-2, January 01, 2002.
8. CIRCULATION

   Christiaan Neethling Barnard

   1922-2001

   David K.C. Cooper and Denton A. Cooley

9. BMJ. 2001 Dec 22; 323(7327): 1478–1480.

   PMCID: PMC1121917. PMID: 11751363

   Christiaan Barnard: his first transplants and their impact on concepts of death

   Raymond Hoffenberg, retired physician
10. Cohn LH (May 2003). "Fifty years of open-heart surgery". Circulation. 107 (17): 2168–70. PMID 12732590.
11. The History of the Heart

    web.stanford.edu › earlysciencelab › body › heartpages
12. Altman, Lawrence K. (3 September 2001). "Christiaan Barnard, 78, Surgeon For First Heart Transplant, Dies". The New York Times.
13. Longest surviving heart transplant patient dies at 73.
14. www.cardiomyopathy.org › latest-news › post › 166-lo ...
15. Isabella's Story | Patient Stories | NewYork-Presbyterian
16. www.nyp.org › patient-stories › patient-story-isabella
17. Heart Transplantation in Asia

    Hae-Young Lee, Byung-Hee Oh
18. JSTAGE.. JAPAN SCIENCE AND TECHNOLOGY JOURNAL Reviews
71. Heart transplant in India: Lessons learned Airan B, Singh SP ...

    www.j-pcs.org › article

    by B Airan – 2017
72. Indian J Crit Care Med. 2009 Jan-Mar; 13(1): 7–11.

    PMCID: PMC2772257. PMID: 19881172

    The diagnosis of brain-death

    Ajay Kumar Goila and Mridula Pawar
73. SAGE JOURNALS

    1967: Reflections on the first human heart transplant and its impact on medicine, media and society First Published November 4, 2017
74. Fricke, T. A.; Konstantinov, I. E. (2013) Dawn and Evolution of Cardiac Procedures, Springery

75. What is Heart? It is the Reality. - Sri Ramana Maharshi

    sriramanamaharishi.com › faith-heart-grace-reality ›

76. Dr. Christiaan Barnard: renowned surgeon, egoist but an old-fashioned family doctor at heart. Interview by Robert MacNeil.

    Rowe DJ

    Canadian Medical Association Journal, 01 Jan 1979, 120(1):98-99 PMID: 367559 PMCID: PMC1818814

77. Impact of green corridors in organ donation: A single-center experience

    Vipin Koushal, Raman Sharma, Ashok Kumar

    Department of Hospital Administration, PGIMER, Chandigarh, India

78. Braz J Cardiovasc Surg. 2017 Sep-Oct; 32(5): 423–427. PMCID: PMC5701108. PMID: 29211224

    History of Heart Transplantation: a Hard and Glorious Journey

    Noedir A. G. Stolf, M.D., Ph.D.

www.ingramcontent.com/pod-product-compliance
Lightning Source LLC
Chambersburg PA
CBHW020739180526
45163CB00001B/284